Mental Health and Work: New Zealand

OECD
BETTER POLICIES FOR BETTER LIVES

Please cite this publication as:
OECD (2018), *Mental Health and Work: New Zealand*, Mental Health and Work, OECD Publishing, Paris.
https://doi.org/10.1787/9789264307315-en

ISBN 978-92-64-30730-8 (print)
ISBN 978-92-64-30731-5 (pdf)

Series: Mental Health and Work
ISSN 2225-7977 (print)
ISSN 2225-7985 (online)

Photo credits: © Inmagine ltd.

Corrigenda to OECD publications may be found on line at: *www.oecd.org/publishing/corrigenda*.

Foreword

The mental health of the working-age population is becoming a key issue in labour market and social policies in many OECD countries. It is an issue that has been neglected for too long despite the high and growing cost of poor mental health to people and society. Now, however, OECD governments increasingly recognise that policy has a major role to play in improving the employment opportunities for people with mental health conditions. Workplace and employment policies need a stronger focus on worker's mental health, and health systems a stronger focus on peoples' working lives.

A first OECD report on this subject published in 2012 (Sick on the Job? Myths and Realities about Mental Health and Work) identified OECD countries' policy challenges by broadening the evidence base and questioning some of the myths that surround the links between mental health and work. A synthesis report published in 2015 (Fit Mind, Fit Job. From Evidence to Practice in Mental Health and Work) provided a framework for better policy and a range of promising policy examples from OECD countries, which fulfil the criteria of the proposed framework.

This report on New Zealand is one a series of reports that looks at how selected OECD countries address mental health and work policy challenges. Through the lens of mental health, it discusses the transition from education to employment, workplace policies and practices, employment services for those seeking a job, the drift into long-term sickness and permanent disability, and the capability and capacity of the health system.

This is the first report reviewing policies against the OECD Council Recommendation on Integrated Mental Health, Skills and Work Policy. This recommendation was endorsed by health and employment ministers from all OECD countries, including New Zealand, in early 2016. The other reports in this series which were prepared before 2016 consider the situations in Australia, Austria, Belgium, Denmark, the Netherlands, Norway, Sweden, Switzerland, and the United Kingdom.

At the time of completing this review, the New Zealand Government Inquiry into Mental Health and Addiction was underway. To help inform this inquiry, the OECD review team presented preliminary findings to the Inquiry Panel in July 2018 and, at the same time, provided the Panel with a copy of a draft report. An embargoed copy of the final report was also shared with the Panel to continue aligning the two review processes.

This review was carried out by OECD's Directorate for Employment, Labour and Social Affairs. Christopher Prinz (OECD) and Helen Lockett (consultant to the OECD) prepared the report, with contributions from Marko Stermsek and Iris Arends, who both formerly worked with the OECD. Dana Blumin provided the statistical work and Katerina Kodlova provided project assistance. The report includes comments from several New Zealand ministries and authorities and it benefited from a specific review conducted by Māori advisors to inform the drafting of the report. The review team would also like to thank the many people who participated in interviews in December 2017, as part of OECD's study visit to conduct this report, and the information provided to the team after the visit.

Table of contents

Foreword 3

Table of contents 4

Indigeneity 8

Acronyms and abbreviations 9

Glossary of Te Reo Māori 11

Executive summary 12

Assessment and recommendations 14

Moving from policy thinking to policy implementation 14
Establishing employment as a key target for mental health care 16
Helping vulnerable youth to succeed in education and employment 17
Improving workplace mental health and return to work 18
Prioritising support for mental health in the employment and welfare system 19
Conclusion 21
OECD's recommendations for New Zealand's policies on mental health and work 21

Chapter 1. Mental health and work challenges in New Zealand 23

Defining and measuring mental health 24
Social and economic outcomes: Where New Zealand stands 26
Conclusion 30
Notes 32
References 33

Chapter 2. Mental health care and the integration of employment support in New Zealand 35

Introduction 36
The main challenges and opportunities for mental health care and employment 36
A sustained programme addressing discrimination and promoting help-seeking 38
A devolved, complex health care system focused on specialist services 40
Early access to effective treatment is not the norm 44
Pharmacology is still the main treatment offered for mental health conditions 51
Strengthen the primary care workforce's response to mental health needs 54
Address sickness absence issues through primary care 56
Increase the employment focus of the health system: scale up promising pilots 58
Conclusion 60
Notes 61
References 61

Chapter 3. Mental resilience and labour market transitions of youth in New Zealand 67

Introduction 68

The main challenges for youth and education policies 68
Mental wellbeing in school 70
Mental health awareness and abilities to intervene early 74
Adequate low-threshold mental health support for children and young people 78
Attention to and support for early school leavers 85
Transitions into further education and work 90
Conclusion 95
Notes 96
References 98

Chapter 4. Addressing mental health in New Zealand's workplaces 105

Introduction 106
The main challenges for New Zealand's workplace policies 106
Prevention of psychosocial workplace risks should be strengthened 108
Addressing stigma, discrimination and misconceptions 113
Understanding the link between mental health and productivity 115
Improving return-to-work policies and processes 123
Conclusion 127
Notes 128
References 130

Chapter 5. Social protection measures and employment services in New Zealand 135

Introduction 136
The main challenges for the social protection and employment services system 136
Overview of New Zealand's social protection system 138
Benefit claims due to mental health conditions are increasing 143
Ethnic inequities among mental health related claims are large and growing 144
A large share of clients have been on health and disability benefits over two years 146
Benefit data underestimate the real number of people with mental health conditions 148
The effectiveness of work capacity and support needs assessments is unclear 149
Many not matched to the right type of case management and employment support 150
There is a lack of funding for and access to psychological support 155
Expand the current approach to building case workers' mental health competences 156
Mental health and employment services are in their fifth year of piloting 158
New pilots aim at higher take up of case management and employment assistance 159
Pilots that integrate health and employment services need scaling up 161
Conclusion 162
Notes 163
References 164

Tables

Table 2.1. New Zealand's performance regarding the OECD Council Recommendations around improving improve the health systems response to mental health conditions 37
Table 3.1. New Zealand's performance regarding the OECD Council Recommendations around improving educational outcomes and labour market transitions for young people 69
Table 4.1. New Zealand's performance regarding the OECD Council Recommendations around improving workplace mental health promotion and return-to-work 107

Table 5.1. New Zealand's performance regarding the OECD Council Recommendations around improving the social protection system's response to mental health conditions 137
Table 5.2. Benefits rates and obligations, for single adults, no children, as at April 2018 139
Table 5.3. Trends in mental health claim numbers vary remarkably by ethnicity 145
Table 5.4. There are a range of mental health competency training sessions for MSD staff............. 157

Figures

Figure 1.1. The prevalence of mental health conditions in New Zealand varies with age, gender, level of education and ethnicity.. 26
Figure 1.2. Mental health conditions strongly affect employment and unemployment and improvements in New Zealand since 2008 were minimal.. 27
Figure 1.3. The prevalence of mental health problems is high on all benefits but the share of people receiving a benefit is lower in New Zealand than in other OECD countries 29
Figure 1.4. The risk of poverty is high among New Zealander's with mental health conditions.......... 31
Figure 2.1. Primary health care services funding 44
Figure 2.2. The prevalence of anxiety and mood disorders differs across ethnic groups...................... 45
Figure 2.3. Mental health visits vary by severity of mental health condition 46
Figure 2.4. Visits to health services for mental health reasons also vary across ethnic groups 46
Figure 2.5. People with diagnosed anxiety and mood disorders are more likely to have an unmet need for primary care... 49
Figure 2.6. The demand for mental health services is predicted to rise 50
Figure 2.7. A model for the provision of stepped care 52
Figure 2.8. Consumption of anti-depressants in New Zealand is above the OECD average 53
Figure 3.1. Young people have the highest access to mental health and addiction services of any age group in New Zealand.. 80
Figure 3.2. Community teams in New Zealand are the main provider of specialised mental health services for children 81
Figure 3.3. Most children and adolescents in New Zealand are referred to mental health and addiction services by their GPs or their family and most are discharged back home 82
Figure 3.4. Secondary pupils in top-decile schools in New Zealand perform significantly better than their peers in low-decile schools 86
Figure 3.5. Educational attainment is highest for New Zealand students when they leave school at age 18 87
Figure 3.6. Educational attainment for New Zealand pupils varies by the type of school they have attended 90
Figure 3.7. Māori and Pasifika students drop out of higher education at much higher rates than students of other ethnic groups.. 91
Figure 3.8. Educational attainment and ethnicity play a key role for labour market outcomes of New Zealanders... 92
Figure 4.1. The labour market in New Zealand is strong and inclusive and working conditions are comparatively good 109
Figure 4.2. Work can be stressful for many New Zealanders, at least sometimes 110
Figure 4.3. Permanent employees in New Zealand are entitled to four weeks of paid leave............. 118
Figure 4.4. OECD countries offer very different levels of income support for sickness 120
Figure 5.1. An illustration of Work and Income's case management approach................................. 142
Figure 5.2. Welfare benefits claims for mental health reasons continue to increase.......................... 144
Figure 5.3. Gradual increase in the number of Māori and Pacific people claiming benefits for mental health reasons 145

Figure 5.4. New Zealand belongs to the group of OECD countries with relatively low spending on active labour market programmes and training 147
Figure 5.5. Primary reason for benefits claims underestimates the proportion of people with mental health conditions on all main benefits 148
Figure 5.6. The routes to case management and employment assistance by benefit type 153

Boxes

Box 1.1. Defining and measuring mental health conditions 25
Box 1.2. The Accident Compensation Corporation (ACC) 32
Box 2.1. The New Zealand Health System 41
Box 2.2. New Zealand Health Policy and Strategy 42
Box 2.3. Māori and Pacific models of mental health and well-being 48
Box 5.1. About the New Zealand social protection system 139
Box 5.2. The 2013 Health and Disability Welfare Reforms 140

Indigeneity

The principle of indigeneity "goes beyond cultural recognition to claim a special place for indigenous people in the life of the nation. It does not mean other cultures should not also be duly recognised …, but it does acknowledge a unique position for indigenous peoples" (Durie, 2004, p. 8). Māori people are tāngata whenua (people born of the land), and as such have a different standing than other ethnic groups in Aotearoa/New Zealand. Māori people also have a Treaty relationship with the Government, which has responsibilities towards Māori people, including acknowledgement of their special status as tāngata whenua. Both the principle of indigeneity and the Treaty have been recognised in law, e.g. Māori Language Act of 1991 and Treaty of Waitangi Act of 1975 (Durie, 2002[1]).

The Treaty of Waitangi (Te Tiriti o Waitangi) is an important document influencing governance arrangements in Aotearoa. It was signed in 1840 by the British Crown and Māori rangatira. The Treaty is considered the founding document of Aotearoa and sets out the promises as well as the rights and responsibilities of the Crown and Māori people. The Treaty confirms the rights that tāngata whenua had prior to 1840. In 2010, Aotearoa signed the United National Declaration on the Rights of Indigenous Peoples, further honouring its commitment to tāngata whenua.

This mental health and work report has examined Aotearoa policies and practices against the OECD recommendations for integrated policies across health, education, welfare and workplaces that will address a long-standing and significant inequity, the labour force participation of people with mental health conditions. Within this inequity, there are further inequities, particularly for Māori people. To support the Aotearoa government to further understand and address these inequities, in this report, wherever possible, data analysis is conducted by ethnicity. This approach has identified the greater labour force disadvantage for Māori experiencing mental health conditions.

Where appropriate and in consultation with the Māori advisors, the report offers interpretations of the data and highlights the importance of Māori-led solutions to address these inequities. As the review team were informed, the principles of indigeneity frequently sit as theory because of the lack of clarity in understanding what indigeneity means in practice. Culturally informed initiatives and a culturally competent workforce are a part of this, as is the recognition and funding of a Kaupapa Māori approach to research (Mane, 2009[2]). Cultural competency is particularly important across public services and means that staff "will be competent at the interface between their own culture and the culture of others. Language barriers, differing codes for social interaction, variable community expectations and a willingness to involve friends or families in assessment, treatment and rehabilitation make important difference to the way care is experienced" (Durie, 2005, p.8).

In taking forward the policy recommendations in this report, due consideration must be given that changes made do not further contribute to the labour force disadvantage of Māori experiencing mental health conditions, but rather address these inequities.

Acronyms and abbreviations

ACC	Accident Compensation Cooperation
BPAC	Best Practice Advocacy Centre
CBT	Cognitive Behavioural Therapy
DDD	Defined Daily Dosage
DHB	District Health Boards
EAP	Employee Assistance Programme
ELX	Early Leaving Exemption
ERO	Education Review Office
FTE	Full-Time Equivalent
GDP	Gross Domestic Product
GP	General Practitioner
GSS	General Social Survey
HDC	Health and Disability Commission
HPE	Health and Physical Education
HWNZ	Health Workforce New Zealand
IPS	Individual Placement and Support
JS-HCD	Jobseeker Support – Health Condition or Disability
JS-WR	Jobseeker Support – Work Ready
K-10	Kessler 10
LMLM	Like Minds, Like Mine (anti-stigma and discrimination campaign)
MBIE	Ministry of Business, Innovation and Employment
MH101	Mental Health one-on-one (awareness training)
MHC	Mental Health Commission
MHES	Mental Health and Employment Service
MHF	Mental Health Foundation
MOE	Ministry of Education
MOH	Ministry of Health
MSD	Ministry of Social Development
NCEA	National Certificate of Educational Achievement
NDI	National Depression Initiative
NEET	Not in Education, Employment or Training
NGO	Non-Government Organisation
NHC	National Hauora Coalition
NZAC	New Zealand Association of Counsellors
NZCER	New Zealand Council for Educational Research
NZD	New Zealand Dollars
OAG	Office of the Auditor General

PHO	Primary Health Organisation
PB4L	Positive Behaviour for Learning
PBFF	Population-Based Funding Formula
PISA	Programme for International Student Assessment
POC	Proof of Concept
PRIMHD	Programme for the Integration of Mental Health Data
RANZCP	Royal Australian and New Zealand College of Psychiatrists
RNZCGP	Royal New Zealand College of General Practitioners
RTLB	Resource Teachers: Learning and Behaviour
SLI	Service Level Intensity
SLP	Supported Living Payment
SPS	Sole Parent Support
STP	Secondary-Tertiary Programmes
TPU	Teen Parent Unit
W2W	Work to Wellness
WAA	Work Ability Assessment
WFCM	Work-Focused Case Management
YOSS	Youth One Stop Shop
YPMHS	Youth Primary Mental Health Service
YWiSS	Youth Workers in low-decile Secondary School

Glossary of Te Reo Māori

Aotearoa	North Island, now used as the Māori name for New Zealand
Hauora Māori	Māori health and wellness
Iwi	Network of people with shared ancestry, associated with a distinct territory
Kaupapa	Topic, matter for discussion, plan, proposal or initiative
Kohanga reo	Preschool class in which the lessons are conducted in Te Reo Māori
Mana	Spiritual power, qualities of prestige, authority, influence, charisma
Mātauranga	Knowledge, understanding, wisdom, skill
Mauri Ora	Healthy individuals
Pākehā	New Zealanders of European descent
Rangatira	To be of high rank, chiefs
Taha hinengaro	Mental health
Taha tinana	Physical health
Taha wairua	Spiritual health
Taha Whānau	Family health
Te Ao Māramantanga	New Zealand College of Mental Health Nurses
Te Aho o Te Kura Pounamu	Distance schooling (formerly "The Correspondence School")
Te Pou Matakana	The sentinel tower, a pivotal point with the constructs of Māori pā
Te Puni Kōkiri	Ministry of Māori Development
Te Reo Hāpai	Language of enrichment
Te Reo Māori	The Māori language
Wai Ora	Health environments
Whānau	Extended family and immediate community
Whānau Ora	Family health (a health initiative driven by Māori cultural values)
Wharenui	Meeting house, large house, main building

The glossary of terms was developed with reference to www.Maoridictionary.co.nz and through discussions with stakeholders during the OECD study visit.

Executive summary

Throughout OECD countries, including New Zealand, there is growing recognition that mental health is a major issue in social and labour market policy. Mental health problems exact a large cost on the people concerned, on employers, and on the economy at large, affecting well-being and employment, and causing substantial productivity losses.

New Zealand is in a good starting position. Stimulated by a continuously improved national anti-stigma and discrimination campaign, which was started about 20 years ago, the awareness of the high prevalence of mental health conditions is high. Knowledge that work is generally good for mental health and can improve recovery is also widespread among service providers, employers, policy makers and other relevant stakeholders.

Comparing the actual policy landscape in New Zealand with the Recommendation of the OECD Council on Integrated Mental Health, Skills and Work Policy, however, suggests that policies and institutions struggle to address the challenges at stake. Considerable structural weaknesses limit the provision of timely and integrated health and employment services. A myriad of trials and pilots are in place all around the country to fill some of the gaps. Service use and outcomes, consequently, differ substantially across the country and across ethnicities. The poorer outcomes for some groups, especially Māori people, point to an urgent need for mental-health-and-work policies to be culturally led, informed and responsive. Regional disparities are the result of considerable regional autonomy across government agencies, in turn leading to significant variability in the availability of adequate support and services.

Significant reforms in a number of policy areas over the past decade have improved the situation but have failed to overcome some of the structural barriers. Health reform, for example, has strengthened regional autonomy of the primary care sector but has failed to resource primary care and mental health care adequately. Welfare reform has helped to reduce the number of people dependent on benefits but has failed to support sufficiently those with a recognised mental health condition as well as the larger number of people with unrecognised mental health conditions. Reform of the Health and Safety at Work Act has initiated a shift in focus from safety to health at work but implementation of the new legislation and the focus on mental health in the workplace is weak. Finally, major efforts to support youth with mental health conditions have led to expansions and improvements in access to mental health treatment and the development or strengthening of a range of support structures. However, the uptake of measures is often low, especially among students with mild-to-moderate mental health conditions and Māori youth.

Moving forward, policy development and policy implementation will have to become more rigorous. There is considerable evidence available on both what works and the type and timing of services needed to achieve a higher and more sustainable labour force participation of people with mental health conditions. Already twenty years ago, New Zealand's Mental Health Commission called for an integrated public policy response and a systematic collection of needs, numbers and trends and identified a lack of coordination between mental health and employment services. Twenty years later, many of those conclusions are still valid and waiting to be implemented in a rigorous way.

The OECD recommends that policy makers in Aotearoa/New Zealand:

- Develop a national mental health and work strategy with a focus on evidence-based employment services integrated with mental health treatment. Such a strategy needs to involve various government departments.
- Evaluate the large number of ongoing pilots and experiments in this policy space rigorously and independently and roll out successful pilots nationally, ensuring that services of comparable nature and quality are available in all regions.
- Systematically collect evidence needed for good policy-making, including on sickness absence and on employment status before and after health treatment, using administrative data as well as regular health and mental health surveys.
- Increase the focus on high-prevalence common mental health conditions, with less focus on diagnosis and more focus on the provision of non-stigmatising support. This is important for everyone, but especially for youth and adolescents and those who have a job but struggle because of mental health issues.
- Reconsider the strict and adverse distinction in the New Zealand system between injury (which is well covered) and illness (which is not well covered), a division coming at a particular cost for people with mental health conditions.
- Shift spending from somatic to mental health care and from specialist to primary care while strengthening the employment competence of the health sector and making employment a focus of the health system outcomes and quality framework.
- Improve the mental health competences and responsiveness of the welfare system, provide integrated health and employment services to people claiming welfare benefits irrespective of the type of benefit they receive, and expand these integrated employment support services to people with mental health conditions not claiming a benefit.

  Use the findings from this report to identify a set of cross-government measures on mental health and work that can be integrated into the Treasury's Wellbeing frameworks.

Assessment and recommendations

Poor mental health costs the New Zealand economy some 4-5% of GDP every year through lost labour productivity, increased health care expenditure and social spending on people temporarily or permanently out of work. It is also costly in terms of individual wellbeing as, at any given moment, one in five New Zealanders have a mental health condition. The prevalence of mental health conditions in New Zealand is higher for women than for men, higher for young people than for those of working age, and highest for those with low educational attainment and for Māori and Pacific populations.

Mental health has considerable implications on people's economic and labour market situation. People who have a mental health condition face lower rates of employment than those without such conditions and twice their rate of unemployment. The employment and unemployment gap is especially large for those with a severe mental health condition. Partly because all benefits in New Zealand are means-tested, the share of persons with a mental health condition who receive a social benefit is lower in New Zealand than it is in other OECD countries. However, roughly half of those who do receive a social benefit have an identifiable mental health condition. Because of the large employment and income gap, the poverty risk is high in New Zealand for people with a mental health condition: depending on the severity of their condition, some 35-45% will live in a low-income household, defined as households with a per-person income below 60% of the median. Multiple disadvantages often come together: Māori people have the highest mental health prevalence and face the largest income and employment disparities.

Moving from policy thinking to policy implementation

It is increasingly well understood in New Zealand that the prevalence of mental health conditions is very high and that they have significant effects on people's employment opportunities and their wellbeing, thereby affecting many other aspects of the economy as well, including public spending and economic growth.

New Zealand is in a good position to address these problems because the awareness of the issue is high. Influenced by an effective and repeatedly evaluated anti-stigma and discrimination campaign run on a continuous and evolving basis over a period of over 20 years, mental health and arising problems, in the most part, are discussed openly. More recently, influenced by research and policy developments in the United Kingdom, discussions increasingly also draw upon the strong evidence base around the health benefits of work. This is a promising starting position for the development of effective mental health and work policies. Added to this, cultural issues and multiple disadvantages faced by Māori as well as Pacific people, including a higher prevalence of mental health conditions and poorer associated outcomes, are also discussed in an open manner.

Policy thinking in New Zealand around mental health and work, however, has not yet translated sufficiently into better policies and, consequently, better social and labour market outcomes for the affected populations or, if so, not to a sufficient extent. There are several reasons attributable to this situation.

- New Zealand is running a large number of interesting social policy pilots, trials and experiments, just like Australia and the United Kingdom, for example. But these initiatives rarely translate into lasting or structural reform. Much could be done to improve the evaluation and rollout of successful trials. Many of the ongoing trials have considerable potential as they successfully integrate health and employment funding or deliver integrated health and employment service, and some are being designed by the communities who are most affected.
- Health and employment services in New Zealand are highly fragmented with numerous programmes and initiatives running in parallel. As a result, service providers tend to receive their highly uncertain funding from a number of different institutions and authorities. There are also many stakeholders involved, with limited cross-country and cross-government leadership. National-level initiatives are also poorly coordinated with regional ones; regional actors have considerable authority over their actions.
- Policies tend to have a focus on diagnosed severe mental health conditions with limited attention given and services provided to people with common mental health conditions including most mood and anxiety disorders that are frequently unrecognised, or undiagnosed, but can also have a significant impact on a person. This is visible in services directed at youth (access to which generally requires a diagnosis); in welfare services (which also generally require a diagnosis); and health services (which are tilted towards costly inpatient service while primary and mental health care is relatively under-resourced).
- Certain fundamental features of the various systems operating in this space make better employment outcomes for people with mental health conditions and effective structural reform quite difficult to achieve. Among those are:
    - A strict and adverse distinction between injuries (covered by an effective and well-resourced social insurance system) and illnesses (covered by an under-resourced general health and a means-tested welfare system), with mental health problems virtually always falling into the latter group.
    - A health system that combines general practitioners who operate on a private business model with considerable co-payments for users on the one hand with a fully tax-financed secondary and tertiary health system with a relatively complex funding structure on the other. This creates a situation where many people lack access to primary health care while, maybe unnecessarily, accessing costly specialist services instead.
    - A general absence of early intervention in the welfare system as reflected in the lack of a sickness and return-to-work policy, including special payments to people who are off sick from work more than four weeks. Whilst the social investment approach offered a mechanism to promote early intervention, the way it was focused initially in the welfare system was to get people off benefits rather than preventing benefit claims and securing sustainable employment outcomes. Interpreted in this way, this approach contributed to poor work outcomes for many jobseekers with mental health conditions.

Establishing employment as a key target for mental health care

Twenty years ago, a paper by New Zealand's Mental Health Commission on issues and opportunities in employment and mental health called for an "integrated public policy response" across mental health, employment and income support policies. The report identified a lack of information about the "needs, numbers and trends" of people with mental health conditions seeking employment; a lack of "coordination between mental health and employment services"; and a need for "better skills among the mental health and employment service workforce". This was a very accurate state-of-the-art assessment and many of the conclusions are still valid. Today, more New Zealanders with a mental health condition receive treatment but the significant issues around service coordination and service integration, with a few local exceptions, remain.

This is likely to be explained by the relative complexity and fragmentation of the system, coupled with an underinvestment in mental health services and primary care-based services over many years. Despite a series of health care reforms, New Zealand still has a health system strongly orientated towards, and invested in, the provision of clinical services, with pharmacology the dominant model of treatment for mental health conditions. Where non-pharmacological treatments are available, access is inconsistent and inequitable.

Primary care has a particularly important role in improving the labour force participation of people who experience mental health conditions. It is also the gatekeeper to specialist care where later access to care is less cost effective. Building the capacity of primary care to respond effectively to people presenting with mental health conditions is essential, preferably while they are still working, but also quickly when they are not. For this, a shift of resources across general health into mental health services is required, coupled with a rebalance of the funding from specialist to primary and community services.

The other main challenge for New Zealand is to strengthen the employment focus of the health system. This needs to include employment guidance and access to employment support as a routine part of health services, and the inclusion of information on managing mental health and getting and keeping work as part of clinical guidance and on-line clinical pathways for the management of mental health conditions. Policy action is necessary as it can help to build structures that integrate mental health and employment support services at a delivery and workforce level, and across specialist and primary care.

Primary and community health practitioners in New Zealand are innovating new models of care, with culturally informed and culturally led programmes and support services. As these are grown, and the mental health capacity of primary care strengthened, this is the ideal time to build in training and guidelines around mental health and work, particularly on managing sickness absence and supporting return to work. Similarly, with a focus on increasing access to psychological treatments, including e-therapies, the scale-up of these programmes provides an opportunity to integrate them with employment support services and strengthen the links between mental health care and work from the outset.

Institutionally, an integrated whole-of-government policy framework promoting the interrelationship between health care and the workplace is required. Leadership roles and responsibilities of the Ministries need to be clarified, particularly across the Ministry of Health and the Ministry of Social Development but also the Accident Compensation Cooperation (ACC). The inequitable divide in New Zealand's system between injury and illness has created a two-tier health care system where integrated health services and vocational rehabilitation support is prioritised for injury, through ACC, and not illness. This is particularly significant for people with mental health conditions.

In this context, conducting a national mental health survey is also a priority. This survey needs to gather data on labour force participation and other work and income outcomes by severity of illness and diagnosis. To inform policy making in this space, there is also an urgent need for accurate data on the number of people receiving primary mental health services and the share transferred to secondary care; the number of people receiving psychological therapies and the waiting times for such therapies; and the employment status before and after treatment.

Helping vulnerable youth to succeed in education and employment

One of the main characteristics of mental health conditions is their very early onset, most often in teenage and childhood. Accordingly, strategies to help people with mental health conditions enter the labour market must include youth and education policies. This is even more critical because of the long time lag of typically 10-15 years from the onset of a mental health problem to its first treatment. Early non-stigmatising support for youth is thus critical. Problems are potentially even more pressing in New Zealand as shown by a high risk of depression, self-harm and suicide attempts among youth. The youth suicide rate in New Zealand is more than twice the OECD average rate.

Well aware of the challenges, in 2012 the New Zealand government launched the Youth Mental Health Project, primarily targeting the age group 12-19 and financing 26 different initiatives across several government departments. These initiatives, most of which are still ongoing, include expansions in mental health services, attempts to improve access to services for disadvantaged groups, and a number of school-based programmes.

Together with the existing infrastructure, New Zealand now has an impressive array of services in place targeting schools and vulnerable youth. This includes:

- The Youth One Stop Shops, an accessible youth hub that combines low-threshold, integrated support with referral to specialist services;
- An effective Attendance Service to tackle and prevent early school leaving;
- Considerable resources in schools such as additional learning supports, managing behaviour programmes and school-based health services;
- Various alternative pathways to complete education e.g. through Activity Centres, Alternative Education, Teen Parents Units, or the Correspondence School; and
- Initiatives that promote the transition into work, especially through the Youth Guarantee (for those still in school) and through Work and Income's Youth Service (for NEETs and benefit recipients).

Many of these programmes and services are internationally of a very high standard. Actual outcomes, however, are not as impressive as the rich suite of services would seem to imply. Despite a great awareness of the need to help vulnerable students and although several initiatives have been shown to be effective, e.g. strengthening reengagement with education or increasing access to health care, considerable problems remain. First, the education system continues to produce noticeably unequal outcomes. Māori youth, the most disadvantaged of all groups, still have relatively poor education and employment outcomes: they are over-represented among all groups at risk – such as early school leavers and NEETs (= those not in education, employment or training) – and among users of most services, while also being the group with the highest mental health prevalence. Most initiatives and supports, including some especially targeted for Māori youth, show poorer effectiveness for the target population. This is disappointing in view of the strong will of subsequent governments to ensure equal outcomes for all young people.

Secondly, many services and initiatives are insufficiently resourced and have to draw their resources from several government and non-government donors. Most initiatives are initially set-up as an experiment and many remain in a trial phase for years if not forever. Trials rarely cover the entire country and even if a service is rolled-out nationally, it appears that the accessibility and availability of supports varies considerably across the country. More national guidance and monitoring would be an important step to ensure all youth across New Zealand can benefit from the best available service.

Thirdly, it appears that the links and transitions between services and institutions in place are underdeveloped. This has multiple consequences, including duplication of service, lacking referrals to the appropriate service and unnecessary delays in getting the right service. For the youth population, it will not always be clear where (best) to go and the outcome may be highly entry and path-dependant. Improving this situation will require more of a nation-wide public policy and clearer political leadership.

Finally, many youth initiatives and services lack sufficient attention to mental health. This includes all non-medical youth services but also school-based health services and even the before-school health check done at age 4. This is unfortunate because children and adolescents with mental health conditions see much poorer outcomes later and benefit less from many of the rather comprehensive support programmes and structures.

Improving workplace mental health and return to work

The link between mental health and work and the key role of the workplace for people having or developing a mental health condition are well understood in New Zealand. It is a role model on mental health awareness campaigns, which, more recently, also started to target the workplace as a priority setting. This, together with a range of toolkits prepared by the Mental Health Foundation and the Health Promotion Agency, has helped New Zealand employers to understand and, possibly, address the issue. This is critical in a country in which workers can be dismissed relatively easily and at short notice.

Employer support tools, however, are not enough. Policies and legislation must follow which is only partially the case. Employment regulations in New Zealand are generally moderate, non-interventionist and often leniently enforced, similar to the United States. This is also reflected in policy and legislation targeting workplace health:

- Health and safety legislation has seen a major reform in 2013, slowly expanding its focus from workplace safety to work-related health but implementation of the new regulations is still weak and obligations for employers vague, and guidelines and supports for employers to live up to their new tasks are insufficient.
- Employer obligations for *sick* workers are minimal and employer-provided sick pay is meagre. Public policy on sickness matters is also underdeveloped, and the extent to which sick workers will receive support is highly variable and largely depending on whether they, or their employers, have any private insurance cover.
- Regulations on health problems caused by work are also problematic, as they put people with chronic stress and mental health conditions at a particular disadvantage. This is a consequence of ACC reform in the 1970s, cutting a big

divide between injury and illness and resulting in relatively poor care and support for everyone *not* eligible for ACC's injury compensation and services.

The lack of attention to sickness matters is particularly striking. This goes so far that New Zealand, contrary to all other OECD countries, does not even collect any data on sickness absence; the issue is largely ignored in both statistical and real terms. Since support by the government is variable and often low, support for workers and their employers is generally a function of whether or not they have private insurance covering their needs. For instance, some 17-20% of all workers have private income protection insurance that may provide unlimited income support in some cases and will provide return-to-work support in many cases. Stay-at-work support in New Zealand is offered predominantly by providers of Employee Assistance Programmes. About 80% of all larger firms contract such providers and some 30% of small and medium-sized enterprises. In addition to improvements in policy and legislation, therefore, it will be critical to raise coverage of private insurance and stay-at-work supports in smaller firms; tax deductions could be used to make these systems more accessible and affordable for small enterprises.

People with mental health conditions are amongst those disadvantaged most from the structural issues in New Zealand. Moving forward, much could be done to improve the situation. Special focus will have to be given on how to expand the strengths of ACC to a larger part of the population. Expanding ACC is not popular because of concerns on the financial sustainability of the system but the current situation is not acceptable. ACC intervention is often effective because support is flexible, in line with injured people's needs; it involves all relevant actors, i.e. people, their employers and health professionals including general practitioners; and it includes vocational services and return-to-work support. Essentially, there are three options for New Zealand for the future:

1. To expand the coverage of ACC to also include illness, as was always intended when the system was originally introduced;
2. To partially expand ACC to include at least some illnesses such as, for example, all chronic work-related health problems;
3. To learn from the successful features of ACC's approach and introduce as many of them as possible in other employment and income support systems, especially the support provided by Work and Income.

After all, it will be important for New Zealand to better support employers running small and medium-sized businesses; to better support workers on sick leave and with chronic (mental) health problems; and to strengthen monitoring and implementation of existing legislation to improve outcomes and identify needs for further reform. All of this will also require significantly improved data collection in a number of fields, such as on sickness absence, to make the developing Integrated Data Infrastructure more meaningful to support the labour force participation of people with mental health conditions.

Prioritising support for mental health in the employment and welfare system

Several years ago, in 2011, the Welfare Working Group rightly highlighted that "gaps in mental health, rehabilitation and managed care services create costs which inevitably show in the welfare system, not to mention the costs to individuals in terms of their own well-being"; and that "joblessness is particularly harmful to mental and physical health".

Structural and operational reforms to the welfare system in the past few years have been unsuccessful in reducing the number of people with mental health conditions coming off benefits and going into employment. The numbers of people with mental health conditions claiming benefits is gradually increasing, particularly amongst Māori and Pacific people. Some 30% of people on Supported Living Payment and 20% of those on Jobseeker Support have mental health conditions as their primary reason for claiming.

At the same time, there are also many people with mental health conditions claiming welfare benefits whose mental health issues are not recognised by the welfare system. Survey data suggest that between 45% and 55% of all recipients of Supported Living Payment, Jobseeker Support and Sole Parent Support have a mental health condition, almost irrespective of the type of payment. As a result, supports and services offered for many are not effectively matching their needs for employment assistance.

The strong emphasis in recent years on moving people off benefit, using an investment approach aimed at reducing welfare liabilities, does not seem to have helped this group, which has increased as a share of claimants as a result. The fact that services and support pathways are likely to differ depending on the type of benefit a person receives, adds to the problem; in turn, some claimants will see their needs better served than others.

Two problems stand out. First, there is no focus on early intervention for people with mental health conditions and for welfare claimants more generally. Better and non-stigmatising assessment and support systems are needed which quickly identify mental health issues across all people claiming benefits regardless of primary reason for claim, and support people to access integrated psychological and employment support. The current pathway to appropriate employment assistance and psychological support is unclear, inconsistent and inequitable. Second, for people who are off from work because of sickness as well as those not employed but not claiming welfare benefits, there is virtually no employment assistance available. This issue must be addressed to prevent hardship and higher societal costs and to ensure better employment outcomes. The chances for people to return to the labour market fall quickly with the time they have been away from work.

Where supports are available, they lack a more integrated approach that combines employment assistance and psychological support or treatment. New pilots aim to support people with mental health conditions to access Work and Income case management and employment assistance, or employment assistance from a contracted provider. These pilots recognise the need to integrate health and employment services. Many of the pilots also have an urgently needed cultural foundation. This is a promising development, but services are available to only a small share of the population needing them. Integrated health and employment support services should be scaled up and the evaluation findings from promising pilots translated into lasting and structural reform.

One of the problems in this regard is the relative underfunding of the non-government employment sector, in relation to the proportion of operational budget spent on public employment services. Service providers have to cumulate service contracts from different public authorities, with contracts being very different if not contradictory and always very short-term. This inhibits sufficient investment by providers in the right type of support. In the course of pilots, the biggest problem has been service access, due to funding or contractual restrictions – in turn limiting the success and learning from these pilots.

Within the public employment services there is a significant mismatch between individual employment assistance needs and the intensity of case management support they are being allocated. The latter is often a function of the type of benefit people receive rather than their actual needs. The mental health competencies of staff working in the welfare system also need strengthening. Such training should be mandatory and culturally informed. Case managers also need to increase their understanding of psychological techniques and have easy access to psychological coaching and support services for people claiming benefits.

Ultimately, a national mental health and employment strategy should be developed and implemented addressing policy and funding barriers and helping to build national coverage of evidence-based employment services integrated with mental health treatment.

Conclusion

Policy makers in New Zealand are in a good starting position through a high level of awareness from all stakeholders of the need for action in the mental-health-and-work space and widespread agreement around the main barriers and most promising ways forward. Policy is also moving in the right direction if only, predominantly, through trials, pilots and experiments all over the country which have helped to improve the knowledge base around what can be achieved and how to do it. But assessing systems and policies in New Zealand against the OECD Council Recommendation shows that much remains to be done. Mutual understanding of what should be done has not translated sufficiently into real change. There are many good building blocks within the system but a number of systemic barriers hinder reform and the improvement of outcomes.

OECD's recommendations for New Zealand's policies on mental health and work

Key policy challenges	Policy recommendations
1. Establishing employment as a key target for mental health care	• Shift health spending from somatic to mental health care and from specialist to primary care, and provide more funding for talking therapies, including a scale-up of e-therapies, integrated with employment support. • Ensure equitable access to primary and mental health care for everyone and improve the mental health capacity and the employment focus of primary care. • Develop the primary care sectors' work and workplace competence, and provide guidelines for sickness certification to treating doctors. • Make employment a focus of the health system's quality and outcomes framework, and prioritise employment in national mental health policy e.g. by providing incentives for primary health services to connect with employment support.
2. Helping vulnerable youth to succeed in education and employment	• Step up teachers' mental health competence and address bullying at school more rigorously. • Ensure that comprehensive school-based mental health services are available for all students. • Ensure that adequately equipped and easily accessible Youth One Stop Shops operate in all regions, with comparable service quality. • Resource Youth Primary Mental Health Services adequately and enable them to provide common interventions (such as talking and e-therapies).

Key policy challenges	Policy recommendations
3. Improving workplace mental health and return to work	• Strengthen employer support and obligations to better enforce the health and safety at work act; and increase WorkSafe's mental health competence, its enforcement power and its resources. • Develop a sickness absence policy including collection of absence data; a longer sick-pay period; and an effective return-to-work strategy. • Provide financial incentives for smaller firms to get income protection insurance and to contract an Employee Assistance Programme provider.
4. Prioritising support for mental health in the employment and welfare system	• Consider expanding ACC to cover illness, fully or partially, or replicate the comprehensive ACC approach in other parts of the (welfare) system. • Assess claimants' (mental) health needs quickly irrespective of the type of benefit and primary reason for a claim to ensure effective matching of needs and services. • Provide access to fully integrated psychological and employment support and expand services to people with mental health conditions not claiming a benefit (be they off sick or inactive). • Further improve mental health and cultural competence of welfare staff and improve ease of case managers' access to mental health advisors. • Coordinate service procurement; elongate service contracts to ensure service quality investment; provide incentives for the provision of evidence-based and post-placement employment support.
5. Moving from policy thinking to policy implementation	• Set up a mental health and employment strategy with focus on evidence-based employment service integrated with mental health treatment. • Rigorously evaluate ongoing pilots and trials and their impact on education and employment outcomes and roll out successful pilots nationally to ensure comparable service is available in all regions. • Systematically collect evidence needed for good policy-making, through administrative data as well as regular health and mental health surveys. • Increase the focus on high-prevalence common mental health conditions, with an emphasis on non-stigmatising support rather than diagnosis.

Chapter 1. Mental health and work challenges in New Zealand

This chapter highlights the challenges New Zealand faces in the area of mental health and work. It offers an overview of the labour market outcomes of people with mental health conditions in New Zealand compared with other OECD countries, and looks at their economic well-being. The chapter also examines differences in outcomes by ethnicity and discusses the definition of mental health and the data sources used in this report.

Mental health conditions present major challenges to the functioning of labour markets and social policies in OECD countries, directly affecting a range of policy areas including youth and education policy, health policy, workplace policy, and employment and welfare policy. Mental health is closely linked with well-being and quality of life and can affect education, employability and performance at work. Yet countries have so far failed to identify and address problems adequately. This is a reflection of the widespread discrimination attached to mental health even though society pays a high price.[1]

Defining and measuring mental health

This report considers as mental ill health any condition that has crossed a clinical threshold criterion, drawing on definitions used by psychiatric classification systems such as ICD-10, the International Statistical Classification of Diseases and Related Health Problems.[2] At any given point in time, some 20-25% of the working-age population in the average OECD country has a mental health condition such defined (see Box 1.1), with lifetime prevalence that can be as high as 40-50%.

In New Zealand, the prevalence of mental health conditions varies considerable with the person's socio-economic characteristics: like in all OECD countries, women and people with low levels of educational attainment are more likely to report mental health problems than their peers (Figure 1.1). The age gradient is also strong and in line with those in most other OECD countries where prevalence tends to be higher in younger age groups (OECD, 2012[1]). Ethnicity also has a considerable impact: Pacific Islander and especially Māori populations have a high prevalence of mental health conditions whereas prevalence is low in the Asian population; New Zealand Europeans have average rates. This suggests policy needs to have a special lens on ethnicity as well as on educational group. Young and low-skilled Māori people seem especially vulnerable in this regard.

Understanding some key attributes of mental ill health is critical for devising good policies. These attributes include its onset at an early age; its varying degrees of severity; its persistent, often chronic nature; the high rates of recurrence; and the frequent co-occurrence with physical or other mental illnesses, and substance use disorders. The more serious and enduring the illness, the greater the person's degree of disability and the greater the impact on their capacity to work. Mental illness of any type can be severe, persistent and co-morbid. Most mental health conditions fall into the category mild-to-moderate, especially a majority of mood and anxiety disorders, which can be enough to affect people's performance in the workplace, their employment prospects and, more widely, their place in the labour market.

One important challenge policy makers must address or take into account is the high rate of non-awareness, non-disclosure, and non-identification of mental ill health, all of which spring from the stigma that attaches to it. Indeed, it is not always clear whether more and earlier identification always improves outcomes or, on the contrary, can contribute to labelling and discrimination, thereby risking worse outcomes. The inference is that reaching out to persons with mental health conditions is what matters: policies that detect but do not openly label mental illness will often work best, especially for young people as early diagnosing and labelling can promote life in a sick role.

Box 1.1. Defining and measuring mental health conditions

A mental health condition is a condition meeting a set of clinical criteria that constitute a threshold. When it crosses that threshold, it becomes a clinical disorder diagnosed accordingly. Threshold criteria are drawn up by psychiatric classification systems like ICD-10, Tenth Revision of the International Classification of Diseases, in use since the mid-1990s. (The 11th revision is scheduled for release in 2018.)

Administrative data generally include a classification code that denotes how a patient or benefit recipient has been diagnosed. Codes are based on ICD-10 and so attest that there is a mental disorder that can be identified. However, administrative data do not include detailed information on an individual's social and economic status and cover only a fraction of all people with a mental health condition.

Survey data can provide a wealth of information on socio-economic variables, while usually including only subjective assessments of the mental health status of the people surveyed. Surveys can measure the existence of a mental health condition through an instrument consisting of a set of questions on feelings and moods such as irritability, sleeplessness, hopelessness, or worthlessness. For the purposes of this work, the OECD drew on consistent findings from epidemiological research to classify the 20% of the population with the highest values (measured by a mental health instrument in a country's population survey) as having a mental disorder in a clinical sense. The top 5% of values denote "severe" conditions and the remaining 15% indicate "mild-to-moderate" or "common" conditions.

The term mental health condition is used throughout this report, to refer to people with mental illnesses, mental ill health, or mental disorders. This includes people who have had formal diagnosis, or people who through administrative surveys are in the top 20% on validated instruments to measure mental distress, as outlined above.

This methodology allows comparisons across different mental health instruments used in different surveys and countries. OECD (2012[11]) offers a description and explanation of this approach and its possible implications. Importantly, the aim in this report on New Zealand is to measure the social and labour market outcomes of persons with mental health conditions, not the prevalence of mental disorders as such. To that end, the report takes data from a number of surveys:

- The *New Zealand Health Survey* for the year 2016/17 that uses the Kessler Psychological Distress Scale (K10) to identify the mental health status of the surveyed population. K10 uses a 10-item questionnaire on emotional states experienced in the previous 30 days. Each question has a response scale going from 1 to 5 ("1" meaning none of the time and "5" meaning all of the time). The final score which rates the respondents' psychological distress ranges from 10 (no mental health condition) to 50 (very severe condition).
- The *General Social Survey* 2008, 2010, 2012 and 2014 which measures the mental health status of the respondents with the mental health and vitality items from the Short Form General Health Survey, known as SF 12 scale, which was developed to measure the quality of life and health. The mental health and vitality questions are similar in nature to the questions used by K10 and use the same scale from 1 to 5.

Figure 1.1. The prevalence of mental health conditions in New Zealand varies with age, gender, level of education and ethnicity

People with a mental health condition by age, gender, educational attainment and ethnicity, relative to the overall prevalence in the New Zealand working-age population, 2016/17

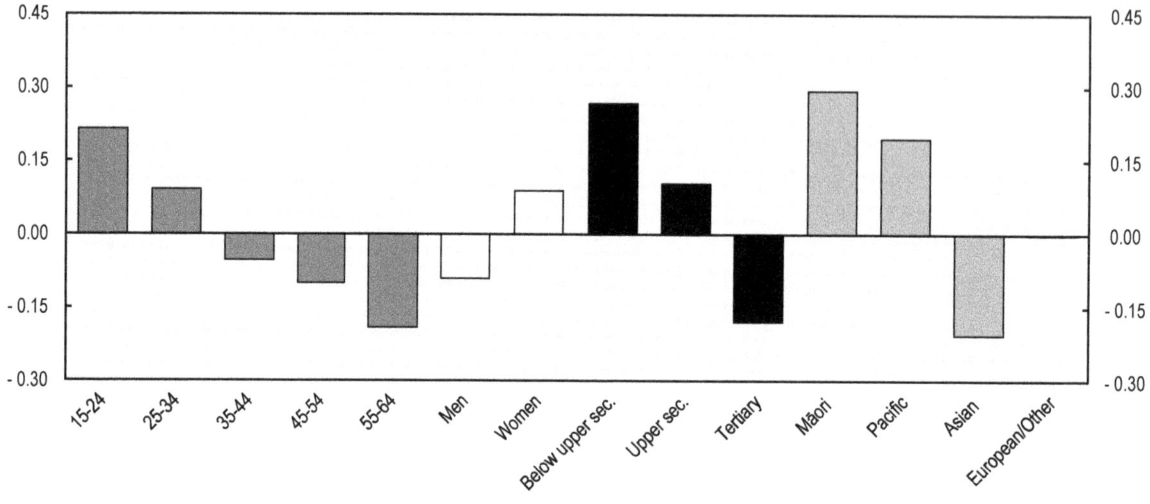

Note: "Below upper secondary" refers to Levels 0-2 in the International Standard Classification of Education (ISCED), "Upper secondary" to ISCED 3-4 and "Tertiary" to ISCED 5-6.
Source: OECD calculations based on the New Zealand Health Survey, 2016/17.

StatLink http://dx.doi.org/10.1787/888933845225

Social and economic outcomes: Where New Zealand stands

Mental health exacts a high price on the economy

According to cost estimates prepared on a disease-by-disease basis, direct and indirect costs of mental health for society stand at between 3% and 4.5% of GDP across a range of selected OECD countries (Gustavsson et al., 2011[2]). Indirect costs such as the costs for reduced productivity at work account for 53% of the total, direct medical costs for 36% and direct non-medical costs for 11%.[3]

Comparable cost data for New Zealand are unavailable. However, a recent study on the economic cost of serious mental illness in Australia and New Zealand estimates a cost corresponding in value to around 3.5% of GDP for Australia and 5% of GDP for New Zealand (RANZCP, 2016[3]). This study looks at serious mental health conditions only but also includes the costs of comorbidities. Other estimates for Australia find a cost similar to 2.2% of GDP for all mental health conditions if including direct costs only (Medibank and Nous Group, 2013[4]); including the higher indirect costs would likely bring this figure to over 4% of GDP. Given that the cost of serious mental health conditions is higher in New Zealand than in Australia, it can be concluded that the total cost of mental health to the New Zealand society is in the order of around 4-5% of GDP and thus at the top-end among OECD countries.

Mental health problems impede full labour market participation

The majority of persons with a mental health condition have a job but mental health strongly affects rates of employment and unemployment in all OECD countries.

In New Zealand, the mental health employment gap is 13 percentage points; this is in the mid-range of OECD countries. The employment rate of persons with mental health conditions is 63% compared to 76% for those without conditions (Figure 1.2, Panel A).

Figure 1.2. Mental health conditions strongly affect employment and unemployment and improvements in New Zealand since 2008 were minimal

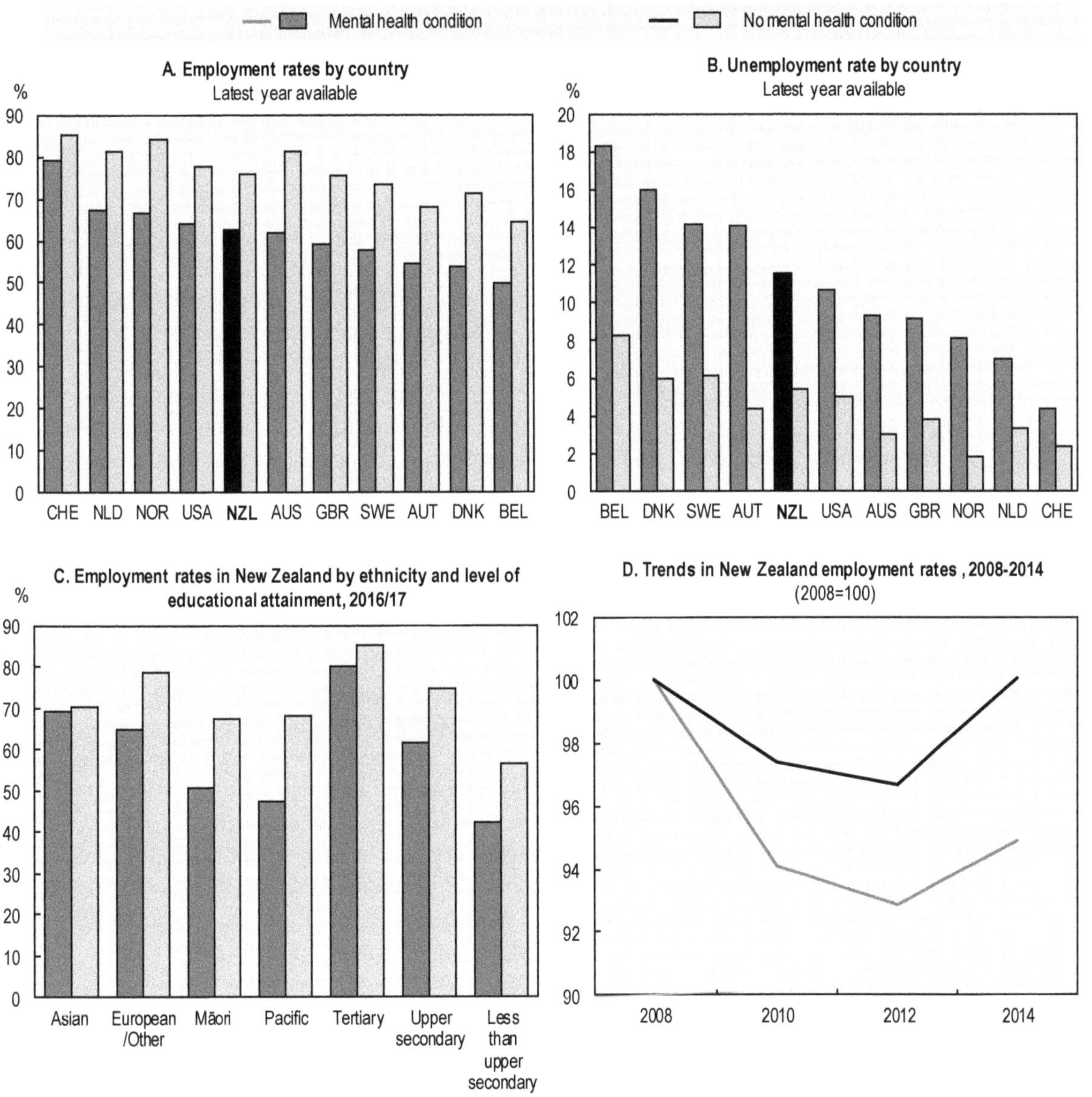

Source: Panel A and B: OECD calculations based on national health surveys. Australia: National Health Survey 2011/12; Austria: Health Interview Survey 2006/07; Belgium: Health Interview Survey 2008; Denmark: National Health Interview Survey 2010; Netherlands: POLS Health Survey 2007/09; New Zealand: Health Survey 2016/2017; Norway: Level of Living and Health Survey 2008; Sweden: Survey on Living Conditions 2009/10; Switzerland: Health Survey 2012; United Kingdom: Adult Psychiatric Morbidity Survey 2007; United States: National Health Interview Survey 2008. Panel C: New Zealand Health Survey 2016/2017; and Panel D: General Social Survey, 2008, 2010, 2012 and 2014.

StatLink http://dx.doi.org/10.1787/888933845244

People with a mental health condition face unemployment rates twice as high as those for their peers without mental health conditions, both in New Zealand (5% versus 12%) and in other OECD countries (Figure 1.2, Panel B). Persons with a severe mental health condition even face a fourfold unemployment risk.

Data for New Zealand further show that ethnicity and education also matter for labour market outcomes. People with low level of educational attainment and those who identify themselves as Māori or Pacific Islanders not only face poor mental health conditions more often than other population groups but also a larger employment disadvantage when they have a mental health condition. Their rates of employment are especially low (48-50% for people from disadvantaged ethnic groups; 42% for those with less than upper secondary education) and the gap with the employment rate with their peers in good mental health is large (Figure 1.2, Panel C).

Finally, people with mental health conditions have not been able to benefit from the economic recovery in the past decade as much as other people did. Overall, New Zealand has weathered the global economic downturn in 2008/09 better than most OECD countries but also in New Zealand, labour market conditions have deteriorated at least temporarily. The rate of employment fell by three percentage points from 2008 to 2010 and unemployment doubled in the same period (OECD, 2017[5]). Figure 1.2 (Panel D) shows that for persons without a mental health condition the rate of employment reached its pre-crisis level in 2014. Persons with a mental health condition saw a much sharper drop in employment after 2008 and a much slower recovery in recent years. For unemployment, the New Zealand story is similar: persons with a mental health condition suffered more from the global downturn. The fast increase in the duration of unemployment for this group of the population has yet to be reversed.

The benefit system faces and poses a number of challenges

What is happening to New Zealanders with mental health conditions who are not employed and how do they earn their living? Population survey data shed some light on these questions. As in other OECD countries (OECD, 2015[6]), the share of persons with a mental health condition among those who receive a social benefit is very high. Over 50% of New Zealanders who receive Supported Living Payment (formerly Invalid's Benefit) have a mental health condition (Figure 1.3, Panel A). This is maybe not that surprising but among recipients of Jobseeker Support (formerly Unemployment Benefit and Sickness Benefit) and Sole Parent Support (formerly Domestic Purposes Benefit) the corresponding proportions are also 50% and 45%, respectively. Moreover, considerable shares of those people report to have severe mental health conditions, irrespective of the type of benefit they receive. This is a big challenge for the benefit system not sufficiently addressed and an indication that maybe many people with mental health conditions if not working end up on benefit, at least temporarily.

Figure 1.3 (Panel B), however, also shows that the share of this group who receive any social benefit is much lower in New Zealand than in other OECD countries; to a significant degree, this is explained by the strict means-testing of benefit entitlements in New Zealand which is uncommon in other countries, except Australia. Among those with a severe mental health condition, 28% receive a social benefit in New Zealand – compared to 36% in the United States, more than 40% in most other OECD countries and even 50% in Norway. For those with a common mental health condition, the share is 15% in New Zealand, 17% in the United States and 20-30% in the other countries for which comparable data are available. Adding employment rates and estimated beneficiary rates together suggests that, roughly speaking, one in four New Zealanders with a severe mental health condition are without income from either work or social benefits. The corresponding shares for people with a common mental health condition or no mental health condition are around 20%. In Australia, for comparison, only around one in ten people fall into this no work-no benefit category.

Figure 1.3. The prevalence of mental health problems is high on all benefits but the share of people receiving a benefit is lower in New Zealand than in other OECD countries

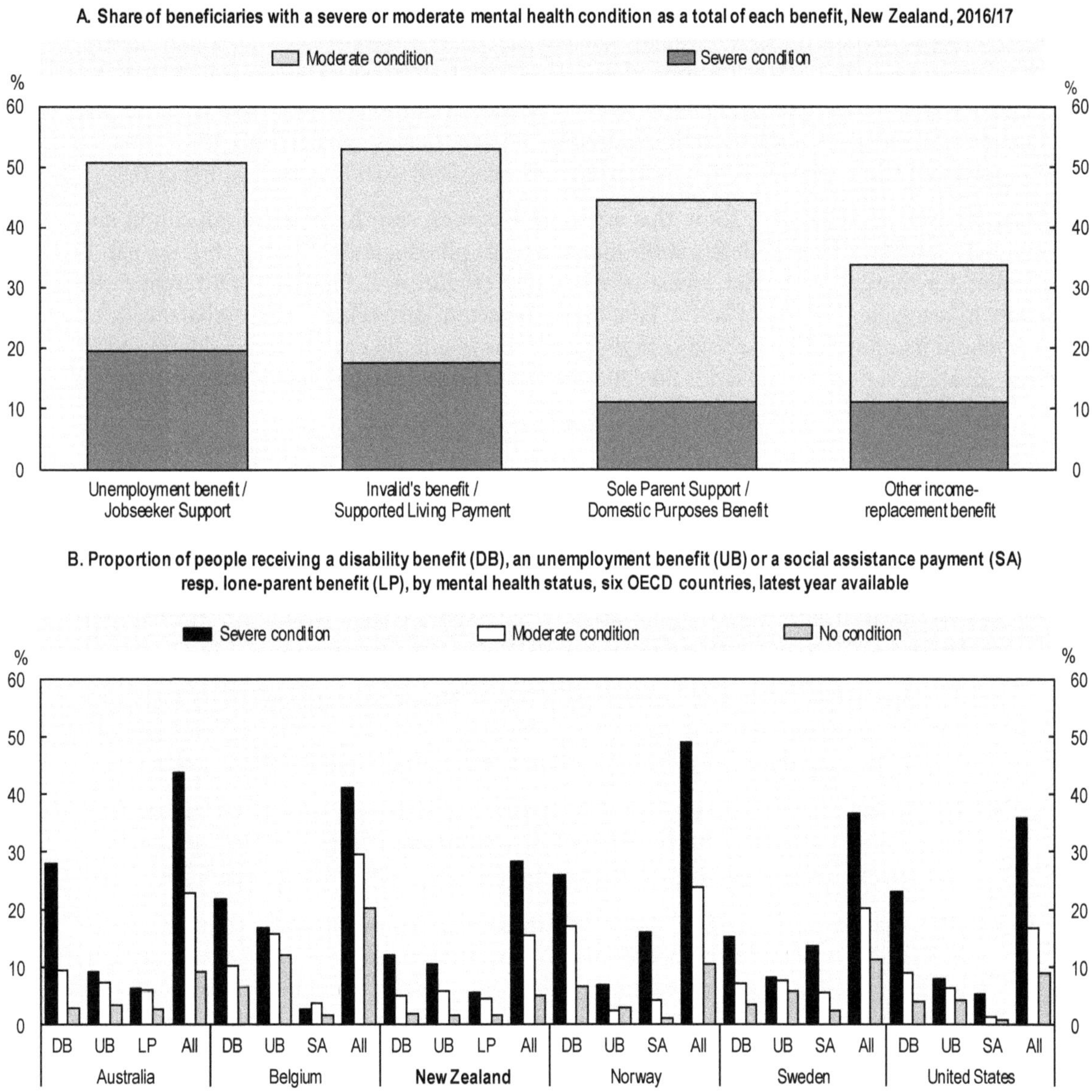

Note: *Other income support payments* include: Regular payments from ACC or a private work accident insurer; NZ Superannuation or veterans pension; other superannuation or pensions; student allowance; other government benefits or government income support payments; war pensions; or paid parental leave.
Source: New Zealand Health Survey 2016/17; Australia: National Health Survey 2011/12; Belgium: Health Interview Survey 2008; Norway: Level of Living and Health Survey 2008; Sweden: Living Conditions Survey 2009/10 and the United States: National Health Interview Survey 2008.

StatLink http://dx.doi.org/10.1787/888933845263

Mental health conditions strongly affect people's economic well-being

Not having one's own income and not being entitled to social benefits implies that a person depends on the income of others, or on own and others' wealth. Income of other household members lifts the income of those in the no work-no benefit group, but it does so to an inadequate extent. As a result, people with a mental health condition face a much higher risk of poverty than the general population. In New Zealand, 45% of the population with severe mental health conditions live in a low-income household, compared to 35% of those with mild-to-moderate mental health conditions and 20% of those without any condition. These rates are higher than in other OECD countries except the United Kingdom: in New Zealand, poverty risks are generally very high and on top, the poverty gap by mental health status is particularly large (Figure 1.4, Panel A). Personal income of New Zealanders with a severe condition is less than 75% of the income of their peers without such condition – a share that is considerably lower than in European OECD countries with a more generous benefit system (Figure 1.4, Panel B).

Data for New Zealand also show that personal incomes vary by level of education and ethnicity. Mental ill health deteriorates the income of all educational groups but the gap is smaller for those with higher levels of education (Figure 1.4, Panel C). Differences by ethnicity suggest that for Pacific Islanders, expected differences are outbalanced by household income and household composition. This is not the case for those identified as New Zealand European or Māori; the latter have the largest mental health income gap.

Conclusion

This analysis of national data identifies a number of significant challenges that New Zealand is facing around better labour market inclusion of persons with mental health conditions; these are:

- Mental ill health exacts a high price on the New Zealand economy – probably in the order of around 4-5% of GDP every year – as it does in all OECD countries.
- The prevalence of mental health conditions in New Zealand tends to be higher for women than for men, and higher for young people than for those of working-age. It is highest for those with low education and for Māori and Pacific Islanders.
- People with poor mental health face lower rates of employment and higher rates of unemployment than those without mental health problems. The employment and unemployment gap is especially large for those with a severe condition.
- As a consequence, roughly half of all those who receive a social benefit have an identifiable mental health condition. However, partly because of means testing of all benefits, the share of persons with mental health conditions who receive a social benefit is lower in New Zealand than in is in other OECD countries.
- As a consequence of the significant employment and income gap, the poverty risk is very high in New Zealand for all people more generally and especially for those with mental health conditions.
- Multiple disadvantages often come together: the Māori population has the highest mental health prevalence while at the same time facing the largest income and employment disparities.

Figure 1.4. The risk of poverty is high among New Zealander's with mental health conditions

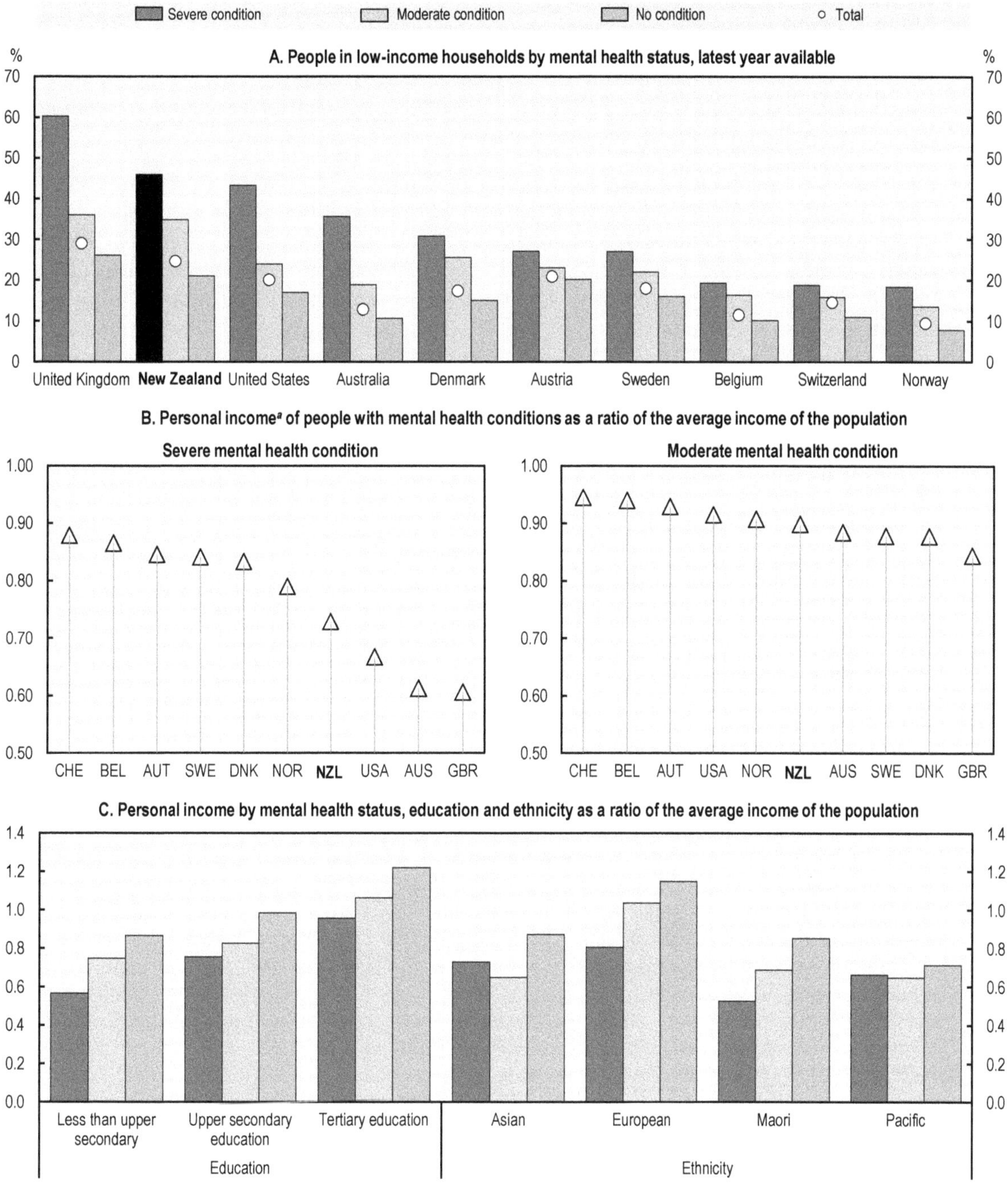

Note: Per-person net income adjusted for household size. For Australia, Denmark and the United Kingdom data refer to gross income. Net-income based data from the 2006 Health Survey for England (HSE) confirm the high poverty risk, even higher than in the United States. The low-income threshold for determining the risk of poverty is 60% of median income.

Source: National health surveys. Australia: National Health Survey 2011-12; Austria: Health Interview Survey 2006-07; Belgium: Health Interview Survey 2008; Denmark: National Health Interview Survey 2005; New Zealand: General Social Survey, 2014; Norway: Level of Living and Health Survey 2008; Sweden: Living Conditions Survey 2009-10; Switzerland: Health Survey 2012; United Kingdom: Adult Psychiatric Morbidity Survey 2007; United States: National Health Interview Survey 2008.

StatLink http://dx.doi.org/10.1787/888933845282

Box 1.2. The Accident Compensation Corporation (ACC)

The Accident Compensation Corporation is a Crown entity administering the country's universal no-fault accidental injury scheme. ACC's support provides financial compensation and supports the rehabilitation of citizens, residents, and temporary visitors who suffer a personal injury within the country.

ACC purchases mental health and vocational rehabilitation services for people who have a mental injury (ACC does not provide support for mental illness in the same way, as it does not cover physical illness). ACC distinguishes between three key different types of mental injury it covers. First, work-related mental injuries where a discrete causative event at work results in a clinically significant cognitive, behavioural or psychological dysfunction. Second, mental injury arising from physical injury, for example, in cases where a claimant suffers a physical injury during a car crash and subsequently develops a post traumatic stress disorder. Third, mental injury arising from being a victim of certain acts dealt with in the Crimes Act 1961 (mainly sexual abuse). The proportion of the population served under this definition has grown by around 700 claimants a year due to increased ease of access to services.

The original Woodhouse Report on which the scheme, introduced in 1971, is based intended that ACC gradually expand to include disabilities of various sorts as well as illnesses (including mental health conditions) over time. While there continues to be some discussion of possible scheme expansion, the current focus of policy work is on modernising the current scheme and better supporting claimants in their access to entitlements under the current Act.

Notes

1 This report does not include in mental disorders intellectual disabilities such as learning disabilities, and problems that develop later in life through brain injury or neurodegenerative diseases like dementia. Organic mental illnesses are also outside the scope. Addiction and substance use disorders are not directly addressed either in this report although many of these disorders are covered indirectly, due to considerable co-occurrence with other mental health conditions, especially anxiety and depression disorders. Many of the policy issues and conclusions equally apply for people with addiction. However, there are also specific challenges around staying in work and returning to work, which are different for people with addiction; these challenges have not been covered in this project and would require distinct policy recommendations and changes.

2 The prime concern of the report is the mutual interplay between work and poor mental health. It uses a number of interchangeable terms that are general in scope to denote poor mental health: "mental ill health", "mental health problem" or "mental health condition" and sometimes "mental disorder" or "mental illness". It specifies, where necessary, whether a condition is severe or mild-to-moderate.

3 Indirect costs in this study refer to productivity losses and the costs of social benefits. Direct medical costs include goods and services related to the prevention, diagnosis, and treatment of a disorder. Direct non-medical costs are all other goods and services pertaining to a mental disorder, e.g. social services.

References

Durie, M. (2002), "Universal provision, indigeneity and the Treaty of Waitangi", *Victoria University Wellington Law Review*, Vol. 33, https://heinonline.org/hol-cgi-bin/get_pdf.cgi?handle=hein.journals/vuwlr33&section=31 (accessed on 12 October 2018). [8]

Gustavsson, A. et al. (2011), "Cost of disorders of the brain in Europe 2010.", *European neuropsychopharmacology : the journal of the European College of Neuropsychopharmacology*, Vol. 21/10, pp. 718-79, http://dx.doi.org/10.1016/j.euroneuro.2011.08.008. [2]

Mane, J. (2009), "Kaupapa Māori: A community approach", *MAI Review*, Vol. 3/1, http://review.mai.ac.nz (accessed on 12 October 2018). [7]

Medibank and Nous Group (2013), *The Case for Mental Health Reform in Australia: A Review of Expenditure and System Design*, Medibank Private Limited and Nous Group, https://www.medibank.com.au/client/documents/pdfs/the_case_for_mental_health_reform_in_australia.pdf (accessed on 05 June 2018). [4]

OECD (2017), *Back to Work: New Zealand: Improving the Re-employment Prospects of Displaced Workers*, Back to Work, OECD Publishing, Paris, http://dx.doi.org/10.1787/9789264264434-en. [5]

OECD (2015), *Fit Mind, Fit Job: From Evidence to Practice in Mental Health and Work*, Mental Health and Work, OECD Publishing, Paris, http://dx.doi.org/10.1787/9789264228283-en. [6]

OECD (2012), *Sick on the Job?: Myths and Realities about Mental Health and Work*, Mental Health and Work, OECD Publishing, Paris, http://dx.doi.org/10.1787/9789264124523-en. [1]

RANZCP (2016), *The economic cost of serious mental illness and comorbidities in Australia and New Zealand*, Royal Australian and New Zealand College of Psychiatrists, Melbourne, https://www.ranzcp.org/Files/Publications/RANZCP-Serious-Mental-Illness.aspx (accessed on 05 June 2018). [3]

Chapter 2. Mental health care and the integration of employment support in New Zealand

This chapter evaluates policies and programmes aimed at strengthening the employment focus of the mental health system. The analysis examines how New Zealand's health system promotes wellbeing and supports mental health conditions when they arise, ensuring that appropriate and timely access to adequate services which recognise the benefits of meaningful work for people experiencing mental health conditions are available. It considers how the system provides training and support to health practitioners, particularly in primary care; and the tools and incentives available to address work and sickness issues. The analysis uses the 2015 OECD Recommendation of the Council on Integrated Mental Health, Skills and Work Policy *as the primary benchmark for informing best practice policies in this field.*

Introduction

Health systems can prevent a reduced capability to work and improve the labour market participation of people with mental health conditions through timely, adequate treatment and the provision of work-focused health care.

To help to achieve this it is essential that all health care providers understand that work has a positive effect on recovery from mental health conditions and they can enact their role in helping people with mental health conditions to stay at work, or return to work (OECD, 2015[1]). At the same time, work-related issues can contribute and exacerbate mental health issues. The links between mental health and work are therefore inextricable, and integrated mental health and employment support services are crucial. Policy action is necessary as it can help to build structures that integrate mental health and employment support services at a delivery and workforce level, and across specialist, primary and community care.

Primary care-based organisations have a particularly important role in improving the labour force participation of people with mental health conditions. Primary health care are frequently the gatekeepers to secondary and tertiary care where later access to care is less cost effective. This is particularly the case once the person has fallen out of the workforce. Building the capacity and capability of primary care-based services to respond effectively to people preferably while they are still working, but also quickly once they are not, is essential.

The main challenges and opportunities for mental health care and employment

The OECD *Recommendation of the Council on Integrated Mental Health, Skills and Work Policy* calls upon its member countries to: "seek to improve their mental health care systems in order to promote mental well-being, prevent mental health conditions, and provide appropriate and timely treatment services which the benefits of meaningful work for people with mental health conditions", detailing key priorities for action policy makers should consider. Table 2.1 gives an assessment of New Zealand's performance against the OECD Council Recommendations, and suggested actions. In summary:

Despite the health reforms, New Zealand has a health system, which is strongly orientated to, and invested in, the provision of clinical services, with pharmacology the dominant model of treatment for mental health conditions. Where non-pharmacological treatments are available, access is inconsistent and inequitable.

National and regional health policy and funding levers need to be used to increase the capability and capacity of the primary care-based system and workforce to identify and support mental health conditions, to understand the interrelationship between mental health and work, and to support people to get and keep a job or manage a return to work.

The prevalence of mental health conditions is much greater than the system's capacity to respond. There is a lack of investment and therefore capacity across primary-based services implying that the demand on specialist services is increasing. Large numbers of people with mental health issues that could be supported earlier are not having their needs met. A shift of resources across general health into mental health services, coupled with a rebalance of the funding from specialist to primary-based services, is required.

Table 2.1. New Zealand's performance regarding the OECD Council Recommendations around improving improve the health systems response to mental health conditions

	OECD Council Recommendation	New Zealand's performance	Suggested actions
A	Foster mental wellbeing and improve **awareness and self-awareness of mental health conditions** by encouraging activities that promote good mental health as well as help-seeking behaviour.	Well-established set of universal and targeted programmes sustained over two decades. In 2017, the national campaign launched a focus on workplaces as part of *Take the Load Off.*	Focus on the interrelationship between mental health and work, promote the role of the workplace, target groups currently underrepresented in help seeking. On-going evaluation needs to focus on i) how target populations are being reached and ii) behaviours of frontline practitioners.
B	Promote timely **access to effective treatment** of mental health conditions, in both community mental health and primary care settings and through co-location of health professionals to facilitate the referral to specialist mental health care.	Mental health system focuses on secondary and tertiary care. Costs to the patient for primary care remain a barrier to access. Opportunity to intervene early, for everyone, is being missed. Treatment is pharmacological; limited availability of therapies and employment support.	Invest in prevention and early intervention; improve equity of access and availability of non-pharmacological treatments, integrated with employment support. Change primary care capitation payments to be based on, and follow, the patient. Invest in Māori- and Pacific-led approach to prevention and early intervention. Communication and collaboration between mental health and primary-based teams needs to be considerably strengthened.
C	Expand the **competence of those working in the primary care sector** to identify and treat mental health conditions through better mental health training, the incorporation of mental health specialists in primary care settings, and clear practices of referral to specialists.	There is a high level of interest from those in primary-based services in mental health and work, and new models of care emerging. Primary care teams have some mental health training, but very limited training on the interrelationship between health and work, and limited time in GP consultations.	Provide payment to primary care so there is time to spend on mental health as well as employment issues. Increase the time devoted in the primary care curriculum to mental health and on the link between mental health and work. Expand cultural diversity and strengthen cultural competency of health workforce. Increase the role of Mataora and Whānau Ora providers and the use of Māori and Pacific models of practice.
D	Encourage GPs and mental health specialists to **address work and sickness absence** issues, by use of evidence-based guidelines and by ensuring that health professionals have the necessary resources.	A lack of precision in sickness certification practices. Very limited connection between primary care and workplaces. Limited guidance and training on health and work.	Train primary care workforce to enhance knowledge about mental health and work and meaningful sickness certifications. Online clinical decision-making tools should include mental health and work pathways, with clear guidance on sickness certification and support to return to work.
E	Strengthen the **employment focus of the mental health care system**, by introducing employment outcomes in the health system's quality and outcomes frameworks, and by fostering a better coordination with employment services.	The health system is medically orientated only. Health policy and strategy reinforces this. Integrated employment support is well established in some services, but not nationally. Promising trials are in place integrating employment support into primary care services.	Realign performance frameworks to support people with mental health conditions get/return to/stay at work. Employment outcomes should be part of quality and outcomes frameworks. Incentivise primary care-based services to integrate employment support services. Develop national guidance and training on supporting people return to work and managing sickness absence.

Source: Authors' own assessment based on all of the evidence collected in this chapter.

As a population group, Māori people experience the greatest burden due to mental health issues of any ethnic group in New Zealand. The issues of mental health and work are further compounded by other disadvantages including poorer skills and an unemployment level twice the national unemployment figure.

An integrated whole-of-government policy framework promoting the interrelationship between health care and the workplace is required. Leadership roles and responsibilities of the Ministries need to be clearly outlined, particularly across the Ministry of Health, Ministry of Social Development and ACC.

The inequitable divide between injury and illness has created a two-tier health system where integrated health services and vocational rehabilitation support is prioritised for injury through ACC, and not for illness. This is particularly significant for people with mental health conditions.

The employment focus of the health system needs strengthening. This should include employment guidance and access to employment support as a routine part of health services, and the inclusion of managing mental health and getting and keeping work as part of clinical guidance and on-line health pathways tools for the management of mental health conditions. Community organisations and Whānau Ora providers also have a key role in strengthening the employment focus of the mental health system.

Conducting a national mental health survey is a priority. This survey, unlike the 2006 survey, needs to gather data on labour force participation by severity of illness and diagnosis. There is also an urgent need for accurate data on number of people receiving primary mental health services; share of people transferred to secondary care; number of people receiving psychological therapies; waiting times for such therapies; employment status before/after treatment. This is urgently needed to inform policy making in this area and monitor the impact of changes over time.

New Zealand's national awareness and discrimination programme should have an explicit priority to improve the labour force participation of people with mental health conditions, and targeted measures and evaluation in relation to this priority built into the programme.

A sustained programme addressing discrimination and promoting help-seeking

The pervasiveness of mental health discrimination worldwide is surprising in view of the very high prevalence of mental health conditions. Discrimination makes it difficult for people who experience mental health conditions to achieve their educational and other aspirations in life, including to find, resume, and hold on to jobs (OECD, 2015[1]). Research into the effectiveness of interventions designed to address stigma and discrimination has found the strongest effects in shifting attitudes and behaviours comes where activities involve contact with someone with lived experience of mental health conditions (the power of contact) and from sustained commitment over time. Programmes that are transitory in nature have less long-term impact (Thornicroft et al., 2016[2]).

Established in 1996, New Zealand was one of the first countries in the world to set up a national programme to improve public attitudes and reduce discrimination. The anti-stigma programme "Like Minds, Like Mine" (LMLM) is underpinned by the social model of disability and the power of contact. It combines social marketing with community-led education. Ongoing evaluation has it has been successful in shifting attitudes and reducing discriminatory behaviours (Cunningham, Peterson and Collings, 2017[3]).

LMLM started with a focus on famous people, which has now shifted to everyday people with a range of mental health conditions, and from awareness raising to modelling inclusive relationships. From the start, people with lived experience of mental health conditions have been involved in designing and delivering the programme. An evaluation of public attitudes since the programme's inception found that attitudes towards people with mental health conditions in the target group of 15 to 44 year-olds had improved significantly, especially among Māori, Pacific and young people (Wyllie and Lauder, 2012[4]).

Data collected during 2010 and 2011 surveyed a representative sample of people who had recently used mental health services in New Zealand and measured their experience of discrimination using the Discrimination and Stigma Scale (DISC-12). Of the 1 135 participants, more than half reported improvements in discrimination over the past five years and 48% thought the LMLM programme had helped to reduce discrimination "moderately" or "a lot" (Thornicroft et al., 2014[5]).

Annual surveys of health and wellbeing, public attitudes and help-seeking behaviours continue to be conducted. Findings from these surveys are routinely analysed to provide information to help to target future public programmes. Of relevance are that:

- People are much more likely to share their problems with their family or whānau (85%), than with an employer (20%) or with work colleagues (10%).
- Young people feeling connected to their culture and experiencing a sense of belonging is an important protective factor to isolation and risk of mental distress.

Annual surveys have also monitored the responses of people with mental health conditions compared to people who have not had this experience. People with lived experience are less likely to agree that most people with mental illness go to a healthcare professional to get help and more likely to agree that medication could be effective (Kvalsvig, 2018[6]).

The latest LMLM campaign, started in July 2017, Take the Load Off, focuses on health and social services, workplaces, the media and communities. This campaign should have an explicit priority to improve the labour force participation of people with mental health conditions. It should focus on the interrelationship between mental health and work, promote the role of the workplace in recognising and responding to early signs and symptoms and target key actors, particularly providers of primary care highlighting their role in improving the labour force participation of people with mental health conditions. Future surveys should monitor the attitudes and behaviours of primary care providers, particularly general practitioners (GPs).

In 2006, the National Depression Initiative (NDI) was launched. The aim of the NDI is to support primary mental health service development and improve the implementation of guidelines for GPs on managing mental health conditions, particularly depression (Cunningham, Peterson and Collings, 2017[3]). The NDI focuses on education and help seeking and has a number of components. The website includes an online self-help tool, The Journal, with a separate youth-focused website, The Lowdown. These tools are supported by television, radio and online advertising, printed resources; and telephone triage and advice, and counselling services for people seeking help for themselves or others. It is important that the reach and effectiveness of these programmes is continually monitored, particularly in relation to target populations and key frontline actors.

In addition to these two national programmes, in recent years, targeted awareness programmes have been developed, including programmes for Māori, Pacific and Asian communities, as well as young people, people living in rural communities and farmers. The Mental Health Foundation hosts resources and information related to mental health and mental wellbeing, including guidelines for the media around the portrayal of people with mental health conditions.

A particularly innovative approach has been the newly developed *Te Reo Hāpai* – the language of enrichment. It is based on a project to research and create Māori words and terms related to mental health, addiction and disability, to help people experiencing mental health issues and their practitioners to describe and talk about these experiences. *Te Reo Hāpai* is part of a national movement to revitalise *Te Reo Māori*.

In response to the Canterbury earthquakes, a campaign called *All Right?* was launched to encourage people living in Canterbury to become more aware of their mental health and wellbeing, how to improve it and when and where to seek help. As part of the All Right campaign, regular surveys have been conducted to monitor the mental health of the local population, to inform targeted responses.

Farmstrong was launched in July 2015. It consists of targeted resources to farmers to promote wellbeing and prevent mental health and physical health problems. The resources, including online videos, have been co-developed with farming communities and health practitioners. The website seeks to encourage help seeking, and includes links to other websites and specialist mental health helplines. The aim is to make a positive difference to at least 1 000 farmers, and *Farmstrong* has developed a number of tracking systems in order to be able to evaluate its impact.

Since 2008, New Zealand has had a national mental health literacy programme, *Mental Health 101* (MH101). The primary funding for MH101 is from the Ministry of Health, which targets delivery to specific populations, but any agency or organisation not meeting the Ministry of Health criteria, can also purchase MH101. MH101 is a one-day workshop designed originally to increase the confidence of frontline government and social service staff but is now tailored to anyone who will be in contact with people with mental health conditions or addiction (www.mh101.co.nz). Since its establishment, MH101 has worked with more than 16 500 people. Māori and Pacific people make up a third of MH101 students. Learner achievement for Māori and Pacific people, measured through pre-, immediately post- and six-month post-training learners' self-rated confidence in recognising and responding to mental ill-health, is comparable to non-Māori and non-Pacific people (Malatest, 2017[7]). MH101 has been benchmarked with five comparable programmes overseas, which found that learner achievement and impact was at least as good as – and often better than – achieved by other programmes (NZQA, 2017[8]). MH101 is based on the power-of-contact theory, and facilitators include people with lived experience of mental health conditions.

A devolved, complex health care system focused on specialist services

In the early 2000s, New Zealand embarked on a series of significant reforms of the health system. A recent examination of the health system has reported, however, that these reforms have not been fully realised. The reforms created Primary Health Organisations (PHOs), to provide essential primary health services mostly through general practices. PHOs are funded by district health boards (DHBs) and operate under a universal, publicly funded capitation system, which subsidises primary care for all New Zealanders but does not usually meet all the cost for the patient. There are 32 PHOs across the country. Whilst there are innovations across the country, to deliver new models of care, these seem to be led by local leaders, rather than resulting from health policies (Downs, 2017[9]).

Box 2.1 on the New Zealand health system and Box 2.2 on New Zealand health policy provide more details on the recent developments.

Box 2.1. The New Zealand Health System

The Ministry of Health has overall responsibility for leading, managing and developing New Zealand's health system. Central government set the overall strategic direction, set expectations for service delivery standards and provide funding. Yet New Zealand's health care system is highly devolved in the sense that more than 75% its public health budget goes to 20 District Health Boards (DHBs), according to the Population-Based Funding Formula (PBFF). The PBFF is a technical tool, which seeks to distribute funding according to the needs of each DHB's population. The tool takes accounts of socio-economic status, ethnicity, age and sex as well as services to rural communities and areas of high deprivation. In terms of mental health services, the funding is even more devolved with 95% of the public health spending on specialist mental health and addiction services allocated to DHBs (Allan, 2018[10]).

DHBs are therefore responsible for both planning and funding within health care in their region, directly providing health care services themselves and contracting services out to external providers. The Ministry of Health oversees the DHBs actions by reviewing their spending plans on an annual basis (as a formal requirement).

DHBs provide a range of mainly hospital-based services as well as contracting with local Primary Health Organisations (PHOs), iwi providers and NGOs.

Whilst having annual plans and spending plans signed off by the Ministry, the DHBs in New Zealand have autonomy in terms of setting their own funding and healthcare priorities, in relation to their local population. Under New Zealand's devolved health care system, DHBs are empowered by a strong sense of local voice and local engagement in deciding how best to spend their money to meet the needs of their populations – including those in the remotest and least densely populated areas. This results in a great diversity within the systems as well as (especially for a small country) a complex administrative process.

Spending on mental health and addiction services makes up between 9-10% of the total spending on health services. For example, total health expenditure in 2015/2016 was NZD 15.63 billion (New Zealand Treasury, 2018[11]) and spending on mental health and addiction services totalled NZD 1.43 billion (Allan, 2018[10]).

The predominant focus of the mental health care system in New Zealand is in secondary and tertiary care. There is a ring-fence in place to protect the spending of the District Health Boards (DHB) budget to provide specialist mental health and addiction services to the 3% of the population with the highest mental health and addiction needs. The DHBs also have a budget directed specifically at "Primary Mental Health Services" – worth NZD 26 million or 2% of the total mental health budget. This budget is for mental health services delivered in primary care settings for people who do not meet the threshold for specialist mental health and addiction services. These Primary Mental Health Services typically involve extended GP consultations and counselling sessions. A normal visit to discuss mental health needs with the GP, however, would be part of the general "first-level service" and thus subsumed in the spending on primary care.

Box 2.2. New Zealand Health Policy and Strategy

The New Zealand Health Strategy and its accompanying Roadmap of Actions (Ministry of Health, 2016[15]) state the need for a shift across the entire health system from treatment to prevention and overcoming inequities in the health system so it works for all New Zealanders. The strategy calls for a focus on the person and for services to be customer-friendly, remove barriers to equity, and work better together.

In 2012, three strategic documents were published that set the direction for mental health and addiction services: *(1) Rising to the Challenge*; (2) *Blueprint II*; and (3) *Towards the Next Wave* (Ministry of Health, 2012[16]; Mental Health Commission, 2012[17]; Workforce Service Review Working Group, 2011[18]). These documents outlined the priorities for how the system should function, the priority areas for service development, and workforce configuration needed to meet current and future mental health and addiction needs. The reports focused on mental health outcomes as well as the underpinning social determinants of health. The service development plan 2012-17, *Rising to the Challenge*, has now expired, without any follow-up plan published. Whilst all documents mention the importance of the labour force participation of people with mental health conditions, they are lacking detailed guidance on the system reforms and services delivery models needed to achieve this.

The current government has prioritised mental health and in particular, child and youth mental health alongside enhancing primary and community responses. The government has commissioned an inquiry into mental health and addiction services, which will report in October 2018. The Inquiry was established in response to widespread concerns about mental health and addiction services. It will examine what good work is already happening, and where system-level change is needed.

He Korowai Oranga is the Māori Health Strategy (Ministry of Health, 2014[19]), which sets the overarching framework that guides the Government and the health and disability sector to achieve the best health outcomes for Māori people. It is web-based, so that it can be continually updated. It builds on the initial foundation of *Whānau Ora* (healthy families) to include *Mauri Ora* (healthy individuals) and *Wai Ora* (healthy environments). The *He Korowai Oranga* strategy argues that "the health system needs to demonstrate that it is achieving as much for its Māori population as it is for everyone else. DHBs have a responsibility to: reduce disparities between population groups, improve Māori health and ensure Māori are involved in both decision-making and service delivery."

'Ala Mo'ui is a four-year plan that provides an outcomes framework for delivering high-quality health services to Pacific people. The long-term vision of *'Ala Mo'ui* is: "Pacific 'āiga, kāiga, magafaoa, kōpū tangata, vuvale and fāmili (family) experience equitable health outcomes and lead independent lives".

Primary care services as a whole, account for around 5% of the total health budget (NZD 920 million for 2017/2018) (Ministry of Health, 2017[12]). The share within that overall budget actually covering mental health-related visits is unknown. Recent research conducted by the OECD has identified that the average spending across OECD countries on primary care, as a proportion of the total public health spending, is around 12%.[1] The proportion of the health budget invested in primary care in New Zealand seems very low, even more so in comparison with Australia's 14% (OECD, 2015[13]), as does the proportion of the total health budget investment in mental health services.

Between 25% and 30% of the total funding for mental health and addiction services in New Zealand goes to NGOs. NGOs provide a range of mental health, addiction and wellbeing services, which includes specialised programmes for specific populations (Platform Trust & Te Pou, 2015[14]).

A range of allied health practitioners make up the primary care workforce in New Zealand including pharmacists, mid-wives, allied health workers, ambulance workers and community health workers. However, primary health care services are – predominantly – privately owned and privately operated general practices.

For the size of the population, New Zealand has a complex, seemingly fragmented primary and community health funding and contracting system. Whilst simplifying the system of funding and contracting is needed this should be accompanied by a shift in funding from physical health to mental health (to achieve mental health parity within the health budget proportionate to mental health need) and increasing the proportion of health investment in primary and community services, in line with other OECD countries. A further barrier that needs addressing to support health promotion and early intervention is to address the charge to the patient in primary care, but not for specialist services. Figure 2.1 shows the complexity of the funding and contracting arrangement. The Ministry of Health contracts with 20 DHBs. The DHBs then contract with several organisations in their regions, including PHOs, pharmacies, non-government organisations, Māori and Pacific providers. The 32 PHOs fund and contract with more than 1 000 general practices across the country.

Figure 2.1. Primary health care services funding

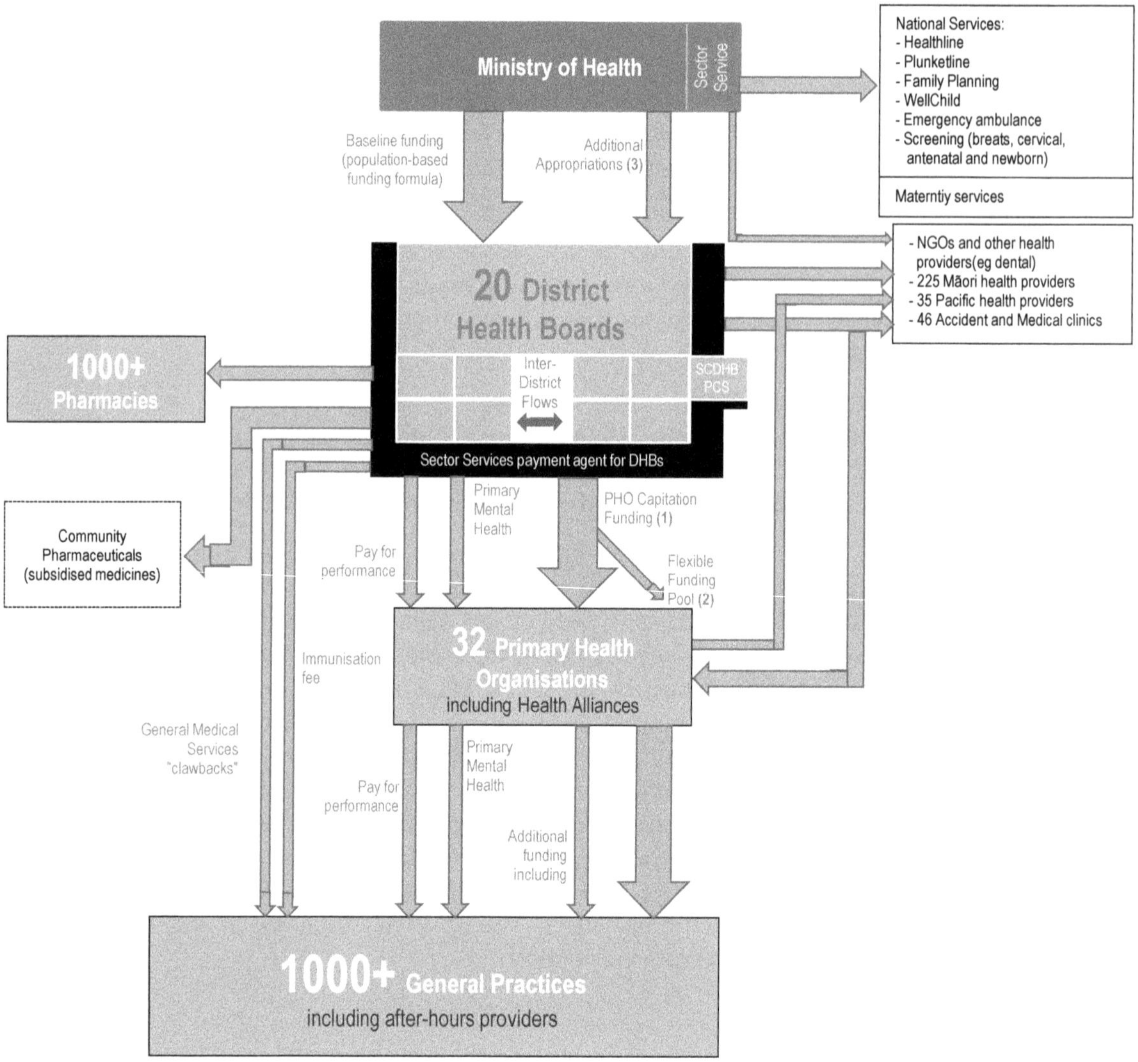

Source: Adapted from the Ministry of Health.

Early access to effective treatment is not the norm

Providing effective and timely access to mental health care is a challenge faced by all OECD countries, as under-treatment is a persistent problem, as well as targeting the right form and intensity of treatment for people with different needs. Thus, in many OECD countries, most people with mental health conditions do not find their way into the health care system and many experience an unmet need for treatment. Furthermore, people who do receive treatment often do so from non-specialists, mainly general practitioners. Very few are in the care of mental health professionals.

In New Zealand, the last comprehensive mental health survey, *Te Rau Hinengaro*, was conducted during 2003-04 (Oakley Browne et al., 2006[20]). The survey used the Composite International Diagnostic Interview (CIDI 3.0) to: i) estimate the prevalence of mental health conditions and addiction in the general population, and ii) identify health service utilisation and unmet need. The total population 12-month prevalence rates for anxiety are 14.8% and for mood disorders 7.9%. These prevalence rates of mood and anxiety disorders are in line with other OECD countries, of between 20% and 25% (OECD, 2015[1]).

Identified mental health prevalence rates vary by ethnicity. Figure 2.2 shows the unadjusted 12-month prevalence rates of anxiety and mood disorders by three categories of ethnicity: Māori, Pacific and Other. After adjusting for age, sex, education and household income, the 12-prevalence rates for anxiety and mood disorders for Pacific people fall to 19%, just below 20% for "Other" ethnic group. Māori adjusted 12-month prevalence rates remain the highest at 24% (Oakley Browne et al., 2006[20]).

Figure 2.2. The prevalence of anxiety and mood disorders differs across ethnic groups

Twelve-month prevalence of anxiety and mood disorders (unadjusted)

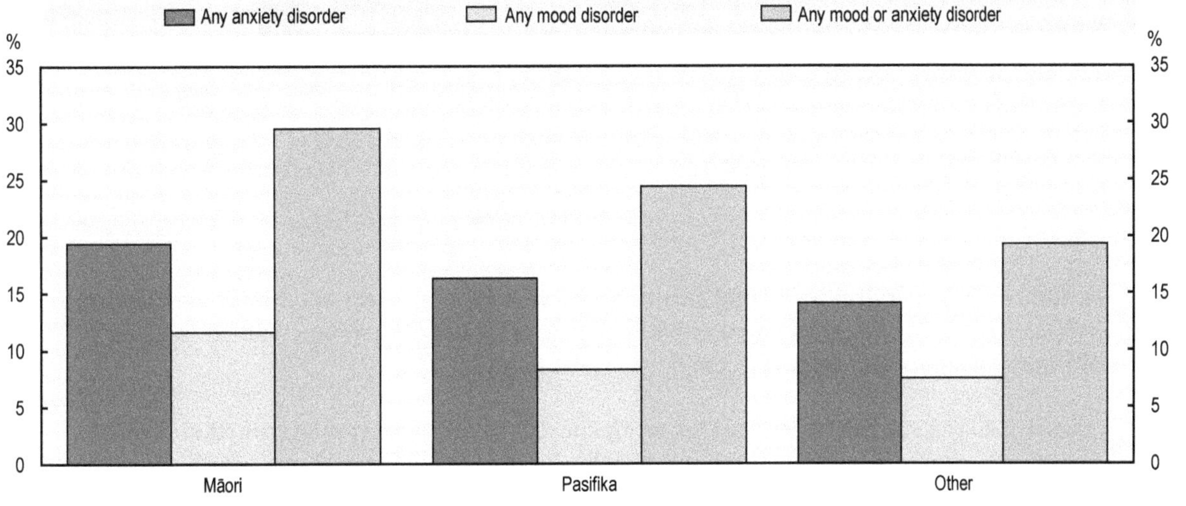

Source: Oakley-Browne, M., Wells, J.E. and Scott, K.M., 2006. *Te Rau Hinengaro: The New Zealand Mental Health Survey: Summary*. Ministry of Health.

StatLink http://dx.doi.org/10.1787/888933845301

Te Rau Hinengaro found that of the people who met the threshold for a serious mental health condition, only 58% had a mental health visit within the last 12 months.[2] Amongst people meeting the threshold for a moderate mental health condition, 36.5% had a mental health visit, and for people meeting the threshold for mild mental health conditions, this was 18.5%. Mental health visits include visits across specialist and general health services, with people with more severe mental health conditions having a higher use of both specialist and general health services (Figure 2.3).

Figure 2.3. Mental health visits vary by severity of mental health condition

Share of mental health service use in the last 12 months by severity of mental health condition, 2005

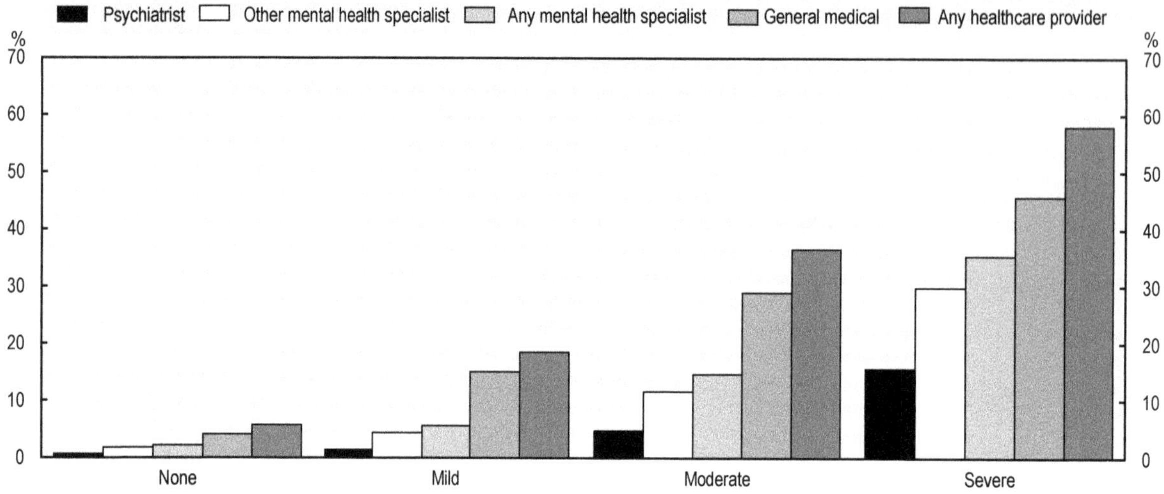

Source: Oakley-Browne, M., Wells, J.E. and Scott, K.M., 2006. *Te Rau Hinengaro: The New Zealand Mental Health Survey: Summary*. Ministry of Health.

StatLink http://dx.doi.org/10.1787/888933845320

Within these access rates, mental health visits were much lower for Māori and Pacific people. This difference cannot be explained purely by socio-economic status, or severity of illness, but was also related to ethnicity itself (Figure 2.4).

Figure 2.4. Visits to health services for mental health reasons also vary across ethnic groups

Percentage of adults with a visit to the healthcare sector for mental health reasons, adjusted for severity, 2005

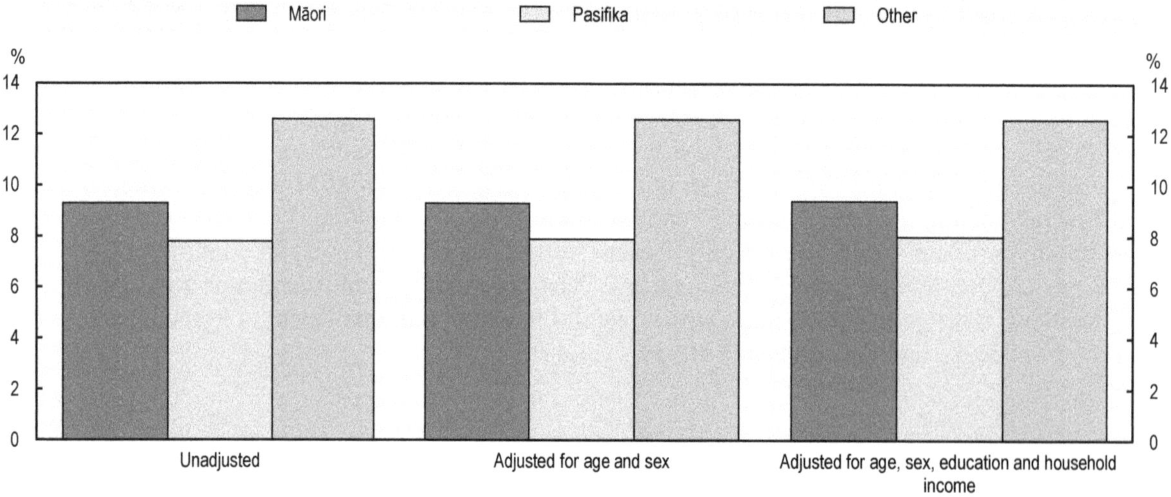

Source: Oakley-Browne, M., Wells, J.E. and Scott, K.M., 2006. *Te Rau Hinengaro: The New Zealand Mental Health Survey: Summary*. Ministry of Health.

StatLink http://dx.doi.org/10.1787/888933845339

A major challenge in supporting prevention and early intervention through primary care is that there is frequently a cost to the patient. This is in contrast to accessing specialist mental health services that are free for the patient. In 2017, the average fee for an adult (over 18 years), was NZD 34.79; compared to NZD 15.59 to attend what are known as *Very Low Cost Access* practices. Primary care is free to children below the age of 13. The current government announced in the 2018 budget that primary care visits would be free up to age 14 and is piloting funded counselling support for 18 to 25-year olds.

Whilst access rates to health services in relation to the population prevalence of mental health conditions are low, the actual numbers of people accessing specialist mental health services have increased from 2.3% of the population a decade ago, to 3.6% of the population in the last year. An increase from 143 000 people in 2011, to 174 000 people in 2017 (Ministry of Health, 2017[21]).

Funding for these specialist services has not grown at the same rate, and the effectiveness of the 3% ring-fenced budget for protecting DHB spending in specialist mental health and addictions services has also been questioned (Allan, 2018[10]).

Māori people have higher prevalence rates of mental health conditions than non-Māori people, they experience higher levels of unmet need, and when they do receive treatment, it is more likely to be through specialist acute services. For example, 6.1% of Māori people accessed mental health services in 2016, compared with 3.1% of non-Māori people. Māori people comprise 16% of the New Zealand population, yet account for 26% of mental health service users accessing specialist mental health and addiction services (Ministry of Health, 2017[21]). This raises the issue of needing different strategies to support Māori people experiencing mental health conditions. The opportunity to intervene early is a particularly missed opportunity for Māori people. Pacific people, people with disabilities and refugees also experience inequitable outcomes.

Culture and health are inter-twined. Health providers therefore need to be culturally as well as clinically competent (Pitama et al., 2007[22]). This is likely to include the use of cultural inputs within clinical practice: for example, the participation of whānau, the use of Te Reo Māori and a Māori workforce. Māori models of health and well-being are particularly important to understand and to build into practice to improve equity of health outcomes (Durie, 1997[23]) (see Box 2.3 for more details).

Data is available which shows waiting times for accessing specialist mental health and addiction services, suggesting that "78% of new clients saw mental health services within three weeks of referral, and 94% within eight weeks" (Ministry of Health, 2017[21]). The Peoples Mental Health Report collected more than 400 stories from people with experience of mental health conditions. A key theme emerging from the analysis was that people had difficultly accessing appropriate and timely mental health services, and for many they could not get assistance until "their health had deteriorated to a point of crisis" (Elliot, 2016[24]).

There are also a group of New Zealanders who experience moderate mental health needs, "who are not easily managed in primary care but do not meet the threshold for specialist care" (Ministry of Health, 2017[21]). This gap is confirmed by data on the take up of Primary Mental Health Services. In addition to the 3.5% of the adult population accessing specialist mental health and addiction services, in the year ending June 2016, Primary Mental Health Services saw 3.1% of the adult population. Together this figure is well below the 23% 12-month prevalence estimate of people experiencing mild-to-moderate mental health conditions (Allan, 2018[10]; Oakley Browne et al., 2006[20]).

Box 2.3. Māori and Pacific models of mental health and well-being

Māori health perspectives

One model for understanding Hauora Māori, which is now embedded in health policy, is Te Whare Tapa Whā, which was developed by Professor Sir Mason Durie (Durie, 1984[25]), to provide a Māori perspective on health. With strong foundations and four equal sides, the symbol of the wharenui (house) represents the four dimensions of Māori wellbeing: Taha tinana (physical health); Taha wairua (spiritual health); Taha Whānau (family health), and Taha hinengaro (mental health). All four dimensions are needed for good health and wellbeing. Te Whare Tapa Whā has become the conceptual framework to support practitioners across the health sector, including the mental health sector, to improve their engagement with Māori people.

Pacific health perspectives

Most Pacific people have a holistic view of health and wellbeing, which means all the aspects of life, physical, spiritual and mental wellbeing, should be in balance. In addition, the health of people with whom Pacific people have significant relationships is also very important. This includes family and spiritual deities. When disease and illness arise, they are interpreted as being related to a breach in a family relationship. Pacific people are therefore less likely to be trustful of unknown service providers and more likely to try to manage health issues within families, rather than accessing help.

Whānau Ora

Whānau Ora is an approach to delivering social services, particularly for Māori and Pacific families, launched in 2010. It is based on the Māori concept of wellbeing, aimed to have the various needs of a whānau met holistically. The aim is to empower whānau to determine their own goals and the means to achieve them, with the help of navigators and building on the strength of whānau. Whānau Ora is family-centred rather than service-centred. The focus is on integrated care and overcoming obstacles that impact on whānau wellbeing and development (Productivity Commission, 2015[26]). The aim of Whānau Ora is to have a strong focus on early intervention.

In 2013, the government devolved some of the planning and funding of social services to Whānau Ora commissioning agencies, these are non-government agencies. This is commissioning by Māori for Māori. NZD 50 million has been allocated over four years (Productivity Commission, 2015[26]). One of these commissioning agencies, Te Pou Matakana, has developed a social calculator tool to help identify the benefits of the Whānau Ora initiative compared to multiple government interventions.

In 2015 the OAG conducted an evaluation of Whānau Ora based on the first four years (OAG, 2015). The OAG reported that Whānau Ora is an innovation and represents new thinking in service delivery. More families are now better off as a result. "The government spending to achieve this has been small, but the importance for the whānau is significant". The report highlights that delays in funding meant that some funds for whānau and providers did not reach them, and nearly a third of the total NZD 137.6 million was spent on administration (including research and evaluation). The report also calls for stronger support for Whānau Ora from other government agencies, particularly the MOH and the MSD.

These high levels of unmet need in primary care and increasing demand for specialist mental health services are likely to be the result of the rationing of Primary Mental Health Services. These services are also targeted to specific populations – Māori and Pacific people, and Community Service Care holders (Allan, 2018[10]).

A recent analysis of the New Zealand Health Survey found that people diagnosed with anxiety and mood disorders were two to three times more likely to have an unmet need for primary care, despite higher GP utilisation, compared to people without a diagnosis. This unmet need was particularly due to cost and transport. The analysis which adjusted results for age, gender, ethnicity and socioeconomic status also found that people diagnosed with anxiety and mood disorders were less likely to report positive experiences with general practitioners (Lockett et al., 2018[27]) (Figure 2.5).

Figure 2.5. People with diagnosed anxiety and mood disorders are more likely to have an unmet need for primary care

Utilisation of primary health services amongst people diagnosed with depression and/or anxiety, 2016

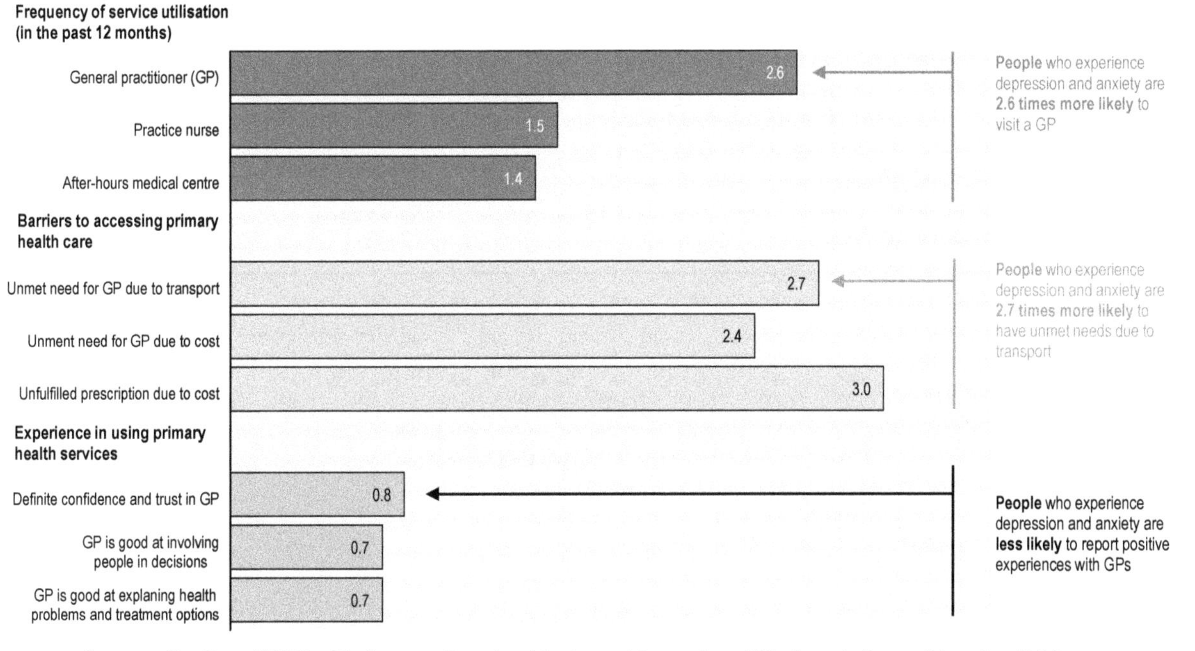

Source: Te Pou (2018). *Understanding health inequities using NZ data infographic.* Available at: www.tepou.co.nz/resources/understanding-health-inequities-using-nz-data-infographic/871 Auckland: Te Pou o te Whakaaro Nui.

In the past few years, several reports have been written about the need to transform New Zealand's response to mental health issues (Elliot, 2016[24]; Platform Trust & Te Pou, 2015[14]; Potter et al., 2017[28]). These reports call for new thinking and new organisation, building a holistic, people-centred resource and services; moving away from a focus only on treatment; and that treatment where it is provided should be recovery-focused, non-stigmatising, community-based and flexible. Reports also identified a special need to focus on Māori resilience and vulnerability and a special opportunity to learn and use the insights from mātauranga Māori more widely.

Interventions are often coming too late or may never come. The prevalence of mental health issues is far higher than the current capacity of service provision, and this therefore needs to be substantially increased (Potter et al., 2017[28]).

Prevention and early intervention can also occur in a number of settings outside of primary care, for example in public health and community settings. At a community level Māori providers of health and social services like Whānau Ora providers (for more details, see Box 2.3) could be a setting for early intervention. Staff could be trained and equipped with skills to use screening tools (e.g. Kessler for mental health, ASSIST for alcohol and drug use) to identify problems at an earlier stage and use brief interventions which could help to mitigate or lessen the problem.

Towards the Next Wave (Mental Health and Addiction Service Workforce Review Working Group, 2011) predicted a significant rise in demand for services over the next 20 years (baseline year 2010) (Figure 2.6). *On Track*, the road map of actions to support providers, particularly non-government mental health and addiction service providers, to respond to this challenge, highlights that the most significant shift in services is needed in the areas of self-help and primary care (Platform Trust & Te Pou, 2015[14]).

Figure 2.6. The demand for mental health services is predicted to rise

Relative change in response by consumer journey (year 2010 = base 100)

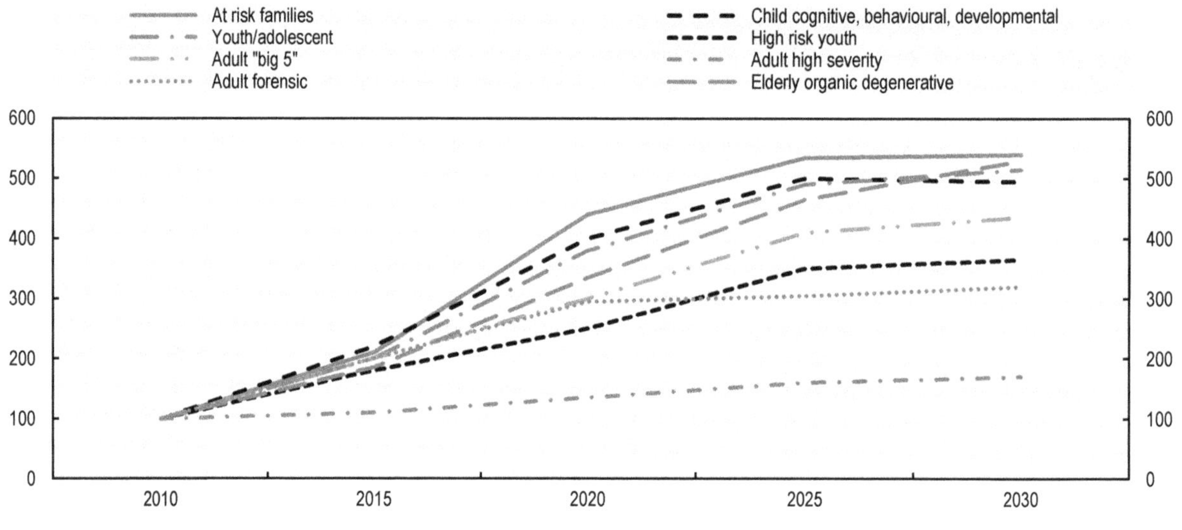

Source: Mental Health and Addiction Service Workforce Review Working Group, 2011.

StatLink http://dx.doi.org/10.1787/888933845377

In the organisation of services to respond to mental health issues, co-morbidities must also be taken into account. For example, 70% of people with a substance use disorder have a co-existing mental health issue (Ministry of Health, 2018[29]), and the prevalence of physical health issues is higher across all mental health diagnoses (Te Pou, 2014[30]; Lockett et al., 2018[27]; Oakley Browne et al., 2006[20]).

Co-morbidities are a significant issue for Māori people. Substance use disorders and physical health conditions are much more prevalent in Māori than in other ethnic groups. For example, the 12-month prevalence of substance use disorders, after controlling for age, sex, educational qualifications and household income, is 6% for Māori people, compared to 3.2% for Pacific, and 3% for other ethnic groups (Oakley Browne et al., 2006[20]).

Whilst this OECD report has sourced some data to assist with understanding mental health need and service access, there is an urgent need for comprehensive mental health data in New Zealand. This issue of both lack and quality of data has been identified by the Chief Science Advisors, specifically around mental health (Potter et al., 2017[28]), as well as across the health system more generally (OAG, 2013[31]).

Conducting a national mental health survey is a priority. This survey, unlike the 2006 survey, needs to gather data on labour force participation by severity of illness and diagnosis, and have a greater focus on understanding the experiences of groups of the population more at risk of mental health issues, and for whom current services are not being effective, or coming too late. There is also an urgent need for accurate data on the number of people receiving primary mental health services, the share of them transferred to secondary care, the number of people receiving psychological therapies, waiting times for such therapies, and employment status before/after treatment; to inform policy making in this area and monitor the impact of changes over time.

The New Zealand population has prevalence rates for mental health conditions similar to other OECD countries, but prevalence is higher amongst Māori and Pacific people. Many people with mental health conditions are not accessing any health services for their mental health needs, and for Māori and Pacific people, when they do access health services it is more likely to be specialist services. There is therefore a large unmet demand for mental health services, across primary, community and specialist services. Building the capacity of primary and community services for promotion and early intervention is essential to reduce the increasing demand for specialist services.

Pharmacology is still the main treatment offered for mental health conditions

In recent years, there has been an increasing emphasis on encouraging the use of non-pharmacological interventions, particularly talking therapies and computer-delivered treatments (e-therapies) (Elliot, 2016[24]; Ministry of Health, 2012[16]; Potter et al., 2017[28]). Best Practice Advocacy Centre New Zealand[3] (bpac[nz]) guidance on the role of medicines in the management of depression in primary care states that non-pharmacological interventions are the mainstay of treatment for patients with depression, these include "cognitive behavioural therapy, relaxation techniques, social support, maintaining cultural or spiritual connections, regular exercise, healthy diet, sleep hygiene and addressing alcohol or drug intake". The guidance recommends that: "medicines be reserved for patients with depression that is moderate to severe, or for those people who have not responded to non-pharmacological interventions" (bpac, 2017[32]).

In 2015 the *Let's get talking* toolkit was launched to support primary care and secondary mental health and addiction services to deliver effective talking therapies, as part of a stepped care approach to treatment to ensure the right support and therapy is offered to the person at the right time (Te Pou, 2012[33]) (Figure 2.7). Another example are the recent PHARMAC seminars aimed at getting general practitioners to encourage patients to take up talking therapies, to get physically and socially active and monitor how this goes, before they prescribe.[4]

Figure 2.7. A model for the provision of stepped care

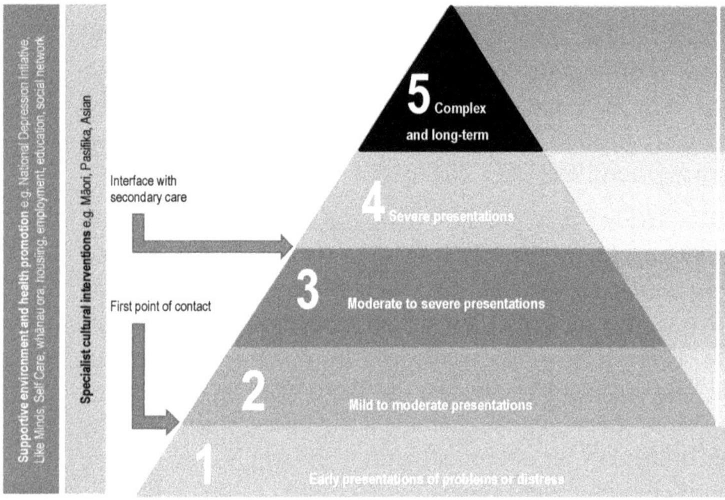

Service level	Examples	Who
Highly specialised	Specialist psychological and multi-systemic therapies.	Psychologists, therapists, psychiatrists and other health professionals with specialised training in psychological therapies.
Specialist	Specific structured therapies including CBT, dialectical therapy (DBT), psycho-therapy, family therapy.	Mental health and addiction clinical staff (any profession) trained in evidence-based therapies.
High-intensity	Evidence-based therapies such as CBT, interpersonal therapy (IPT) acceptance and commitment therapy (ACT), solution focused therapy.	PHOs, NGOs, primary health care and community practitioners.
Low-intensity	Brief evidence-based therapy i.e. guided self-help, cognitive behavior therapy , e-therapy, motivational interviewing.	Primary health care and community practitioners.
Early idenification of vulnerability	Brief interventions including active monitoring, education, information, self-care.	GPs and other health care professionals who have first contact with service users.

Source: Te Pou (2018), *A stepped care approach to talking therapies.* Available at www.tepou.co.nz/uploads/files/resource-assets/lets-get-talking-introduction-factsheet.pdf Auckland: Te Pou o te Whakaaro Nui.

However, delivery models and availability of psychological therapies nationally is inconsistent across the country, and across secondary and primary care, and a national-driven strategy for the direction, consistency and equity of access of psychological therapies has been recommended. Experiences of national strategies overseas, most notably the UK's Increasing Access to Psychological Therapies Programme and Australia's Better Access to Allied Psychological Services component of the Better Outcomes in Mental Health Care programme show uptake increased and there were significant clinical outcomes for those who participated (Bassilios et al., 2013[34]).

Cost-benefit modelling by the University of Auckland, to explore the economic case for increasing access to psychological therapies in New Zealand primary care found that for every dollar spent in Cognitive Behavioural Therapy, society could expect to receive NZD 15.19 in increased output and cost savings. In secondary services, where the duration of therapy would be longer and therefore costlier, the return was NZD 4.47 for every dollar spent (Te Pou, 2012[33]).

E-therapies, based on cognitive behavioural techniques are increasingly being made available in New Zealand, with online programmes such as The Journal (part of the National Depression Initiative), SPARX (aimed at young people), and Aunty Dee. The Journal collects routine data from users before, midway and after the sessions, based on responses to questions using PHQ-9. Data indicates that depression scores reduce for users who complete more than half the sessions, although findings from this routinely collected data should be interpreted with caution (KPMG, 2013[35]). A multi-centred randomised controlled trial of SPARX found that it was as effective as standard care for youths aged between 12 and 19 years seeking help for depression and equally effective across ethnic groups, gender and age. Better outcomes were found when people completed at least half the modules (Merry et al., 2012[36]). The authors recommended that SPARX could address some of the unmet demand for mental health treatment.

Whilst the initiation of these e-therapies is encouraging, there is concern that they are not as clearly linked to primary and community care as they could be, or targeted at subgroup populations, especially if compared to similar e-therapies in Australia (KPMG, 2013[35]). Further evaluation of the uptake, impact and effectiveness of these e-therapies, and others that are developed and made available, is needed.

In 2015, the government amalgamated all health helpline telephone services under the new National Telehealth Service operating 24 hours day, 365 days a year. In June 2017, the "Need to talk?" service was launched as part of the National Telehealth Service specifically to provide a single number for mental health advice and support. The National Telehealth Service is linked to the National Depression Initiative.

At the same time as there have been initiatives to increase the availability of non-pharmacological interventions, New Zealand prescribing data for anti-depressants shows a steady rise over the past 25 years, with scripts per 1 000 population more than tripling from 102/1 000 in 1993, to 376/1 000 in 2016.

Data using the unit of measurement "Defined daily dosage (DDD) per 1 000 inhabitants (per day)", enables comparison across countries. Figure 2.8 shows that consumption of anti-depressants in New Zealand is above average compared to other OECD countries, but still much lower than say, for example, Australia.

Figure 2.8. Consumption of anti-depressants in New Zealand is above the OECD average

Antidepressant drug consumption, 2000 and 2016[a]

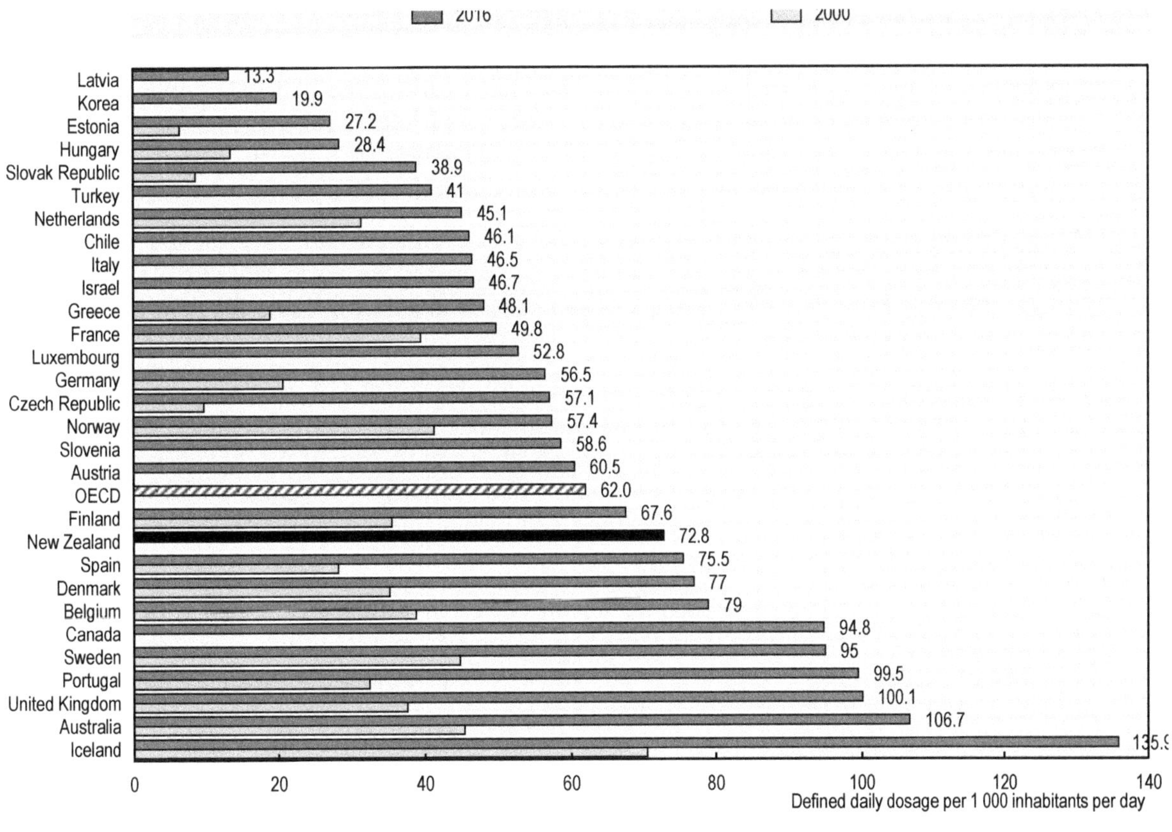

Note: OECD is the unweighted average of the 29 countries in the chart.
a) Early data are 2001 for the Netherlands. Latest data are 2009 for France, 2014 for New Zealand and 2015 for Denmark and Greece.
Source: OECD Dataset: Pharmaceutical Market, http://stats.oecd.org//Index.aspx?QueryId=30135.

StatLink http://dx.doi.org/10.1787/888933845396

An important mechanism for increasing access to psychological therapies would be to remove the cap on spending for these therapies with the Primary Mental Health Services budget. The budget for spending on psychotropic medications does not appear to be capped in the same way. Currently people who can afford to pay, can access psychological therapies, but for those who cannot, they will depend on funded therapy, which is significantly limited. It is also important that there is increased access to e-therapies, but effectiveness of the therapies and their reach and effectiveness to groups at greater risk of mental health conditions needs monitoring.

Increasing access to talking therapies is an important cross-government priority not only in health policy, but in all policy areas covered in this report, namely education, workplaces and employment services too.

Strengthen the primary care workforce's response to mental health needs

In most countries, GPs are the gatekeepers of mental health care. Patients, however, do not always directly present their complaints as mental health conditions, and therefore these conditions remain unidentified. GPs are not only gatekeepers of mental health care, but also the main providers of treatment for those with mild-to-moderate conditions. It is therefore essential that primary care teams, including GPs can recognise and respond to patients with mental health conditions.

As outlined earlier in the chapter, there are high levels of unmet need for primary care services, and there remain huge inequities of access especially for Māori and Pacific populations. Capitation payments based on, and which follow, the patient, as opposed to the primary care practice, to more accurately reimburse providers for patients with higher and more complex needs, have been recommended (Downs, 2017[9]). This is particularly important given the private business models operated within primary care.

Where people do access primary care services, it is estimated half have mental health conditions even if the condition may not be the reason for the visit (MaGPIe Research Group, 2003[37]). Most of these people will only see primary care teams for their mental health care (Lockett et al., 2018[27]).

The GP training curriculum developed and run by the RNZCGPs contains a training module on mental health. The aims of this module are to train GPs to diagnose, manage and treat mental health conditions, help patients to develop coping mechanisms and to demonstrate safe and competent prescribing. The training also aims to build GPs competency to participate in shared diagnosis and management of patients whose mental health conditions need specialist care input.

To improve the management of mental health issues in primary care, the RNZCGPs should review the proportion of the curriculum devoted to mental health to ensure this is commensurate with need. It should also develop a system for monitoring GP competency around mental health treatment and management. Given the significant inequities of access and treatment for Māori people, it is crucial that Māori models of mental health and wellbeing inform current and future GP training.

A New Zealand study, which examined the experience of general practitioners in relation to identifying and managing mental health conditions in primary care, identified that the assertion that GPs "miss" many psychological disorders is too simplistic (Dowell et al., 2009[38]). The study found that diagnosis of mental health conditions was related to previous consultation rates, with GPs non-recognition of mental health problems largely occurring among patients with little recent contact with the GP (MaGPIe Research Group, 2003[37]). The authors argue therefore that strategies that improve the continuity of care and target new or infrequent attenders to primary care may be more effective at supporting primary care identification than training and education alone.

A programme to build the competencies of primary care nurses in mental health and addiction has been available since 2012. The credentialing framework was developed by the New Zealand College of Mental Health Nurses (Te Ao Māramantanga). The framework provides primary care nurses with consistency of knowledge and skills to people experiencing mental health and addiction issues within primary care. Qualitative feedback from nurses who completed the programme was positive, with nurses reporting that it fills an important gap in their skills, knowledge and confidence.

Primary care organisations are also responding to the need to strengthen the mental health competencies and capacity of primary care. In 2016, Network 4, a collaboration of the four largest PHOs in New Zealand published *Closing the Loop*, to articulate a future vision for primary care-based mental health services. This called for better access, early intervention and developing a capable workforce.

There is also evidence in different regions of PHOs implementing new models of care to enhance primary mental health. For example, *Kia Kaha* based on the Stanford health coaching model aims to empower people with long-term conditions, including mental health conditions in the management of their condition. Peer health coaches as well as clinicians are employed. A two-year pilot in five general practice teams in Auckland is building on *Kia Kaha*. Health coaches and health improvement practitioners are part of the primary care team, as well as support workers from non-government organisations. Mental health nurses, health psychologists, clinical psychologists and GPs have been trained on the behavioural health consultancy model from the United States. Practice improvements include formal connections with specialist mental health and addiction teams and improved access to talking therapies. Initial service evaluation shows 60% of patients presenting for mental health support are being seen on the same day. A formal evaluation is underway.

On the East coast of New Zealand's North Island, an innovative partnership between the DHB, PHOs and local iwi has launched *Te Kuwatawata* to improve access to specialist mental health and addiction services, particularly for Māori people through a community focused, culturally informed single point of access. New premises in the community have been sourced, moving away from one-to-one clinician based meetings and taking a group approach to providing services.

Te Hikuwai (Resources for wellbeing) has recently been launched as a resource to support primary care practitioners in the early identification and treatment of mental health and addiction problems in adults. It is part of the *Let's get talking* toolkit and based on the evidence that brief interventions can improve people's wellbeing by preventing mild issues from becoming worse. *Te Hikuwai* has 20 topics related to mental health and addiction problems, wellbeing prescriptions and self-help resources for patients to take away. It is aimed at supporting primary care practitioners to deliver levels 1 and 2 of a stepped care approach. Uptake of the resource is being encouraged across all PHOs, following a trial in Northland primary care services in 2016. Since then, four further regions have adopted it.

Other OECD countries have been developing ways to increase the mental health specialist advice available in primary care. In Australia, the Mental Health Nurses

Incentive programme funded GPs to hire mental health nurses (OECD, 2015[13]). This was found to not just improve mental health symptoms, but equally so participation in employment. Similarly, the Netherlands brought additional clinical expertise into general practices through mental health nurses, psychologists and social workers, and corresponding financial incentives for GPs to involve these professionals (OECD, 2014[39]).

Given that prevalence and access rates vary across ethnic groups, culturally-informed and culturally-led initiatives are needed. Whilst for many people presenting with mental health symptoms, the GP is likely to be an important first contact, for others the GP will not be. It is therefore important to understand and engage with other people and organisations who will be a first contact point. For example, Le Va, the Pacific workforce and information centre for mental health and addiction, has been reaching out to sports leaders and sports coaches, along with church leaders. This is because they recognise that for many Pacific people these groups will be the first contact when signs of distress are showing.

The primary care funding structure needs to work for primary care to provide mental health care, especially for those people with significant needs that, however, do not meet the threshold for specialist services. The funding structure also needs to include time for primary care to have conversations with patients about taking up work, or returning to employment.

The health workforce also needs to reflect the diversity of the people who contact mental health services across primary and secondary services. Data on the ethnicity of staff working in specialist mental health and addiction services shows that Māori staff significantly underrepresent mental health and addiction service users: 9% of staff identify as Māori, whereas Māori people comprise 23% of service users (Te Pou, 2017[40]). The under-representation of Māori and Pacific people in the health workforce is an important issue that needs addressing, as does the cultural competency of the primary care workforce. Evidence shows that access to services improves for indigenous communities when the workforce reflects the local community. Workforce diversity and cultural competency is therefore particularly important for mental health services due to the high prevalence of mental health issues among Māori and Pacific communities (Ministry of Health, 2018[29]).

The communication between primary care and specialist mental health services has been an area that has also been highlighted repeatedly as needing improvement. National guidance and the emerging models of care both need to ensure this communication issue is addressed, and formal mechanisms established.

Address sickness absence issues through primary care

There is a vast body of evidence showing that people with mental ill-health are one of the highest risk groups for long-term sickness absence (OECD, 2015[1]). "GPs need to be knowledgeable about the impact of work on mental health, and vice versa, given that they are generally responsible for certifying sickness and that most people with mental health conditions are treated by their GP". A common misconception among GPs, and health care providers in general, is that people with mental ill-health need to be cured before they can return to work. However, long absences from work increase the risk of permanent work disability (Koning, 2004[41]). Timely return to work is therefore paramount.

New Zealand primary care teams need to be knowledgeable about the impact of work on mental health and vice-versa given that most people with mental health conditions who seek treatment will see only their GP or practice nurse. Whilst New Zealand does not collect national data on sickness absence, overseas data shows that people with mental health conditions are more likely to be taking sick leave and that the average absence is longer (OECD, 2015[11]). In New Zealand GPs are the main health professional certifying sickness absence and incapacity to work.

The GP curriculum developed and run by the Royal New Zealand College of General Practitioners contains a training module on health and work, introduced in 2012. The competencies included in the health and work module include being able to:

- communicate and negotiate with patients on creating rehabilitation and return-to-work plans;
- develop an awareness of, and show the ability to complete, certification documents to communicate opinion accurately;
- take an accurate occupational history;
- assess fitness to work;
- understand the principles of rehabilitation relating to physical, psychological, social, recreational and cultural needs;
- develop and maintain up-to-date knowledge of the impact of joblessness on health;
- recognise the impact of long-term health conditions on work capacity and the role of interventions for minimising disability;
- understand the biopsychosocial model of illness and disease and its relevance in assessing fitness for work;
- identify ways of supporting Māori in their workplace and back into work, reducing inequities that will have an impact on health outcomes.

Whilst it is encouraging to see this curriculum development, stronger links could be made between the RNZCGP's mental health module and the health and work module. The interrelationship of mental health and work appears to be absent from the mental health module, and mental health appears to be absent from the health and work module. It is also important that the health and work module is a compulsory element of training and that RNZCGP finds ways to provide comparable upskilling to GPs who qualified prior to the health and work module being initiated.

Web-based information portals for health practitioners, designed for use at point of care, primarily for general practitioners are used in many parts of the country, these include *Health Pathways* and *Map of Medicine*. Whilst the depression and anxiety pathways mention return to work, information is limited. Similarly, the pathways on work assessment and rehabilitation contain limited, if any, information about mental health. Specific information and guidance on return to work and managing sickness absence / return to work consultations in primary care should be developed and included.

Training and continuing professional development for GPs and other primary care practitioners is also developed and delivered by PHOs, and through some Universities, such as the Goodfellow Unit within the University of Auckland. These offer important platforms from which to provide training to the primary care workforce to enhance knowledge about work, return to work, the link between mental health and work, and preparing meaningful medical certifications.

There is an absence of any national guidelines or training on return to work practices and managing sickness absence. For example online decision support tools, such as Health Pathways, where the treatment pathways for depression and anxiety refer to return to work, could be considerably strengthened to include recommended guidance for health practitioners to manage sickness absence and mental health and work conversations. In Sweden, for example the Swedish National Board of Health and Welfare developed and published illness-specific guidelines for about 100 major illnesses, including many mental health conditions, which included anticipated return to work outcomes, and average sickness absence time periods. An evaluation found that 76% of GPs were using the guidelines and that duration of sickness absence was reduced. Similarly, the Netherlands also developed national guidelines to help GPs discuss sickness absence and plan and support return to work, or commencement of work. These guidelines included information on other agencies to involve (OECD, 2015[1]).

Collaborative work between the Canterbury Chamber of Commerce, employers and Pegasus Health PHO aims to strengthen the links between primary care and local employers, and support better management of employee sickness absence.

Increase the employment focus of the health system: scale up promising pilots

Clinical treatment alone does not produce good work outcomes for people with mental health conditions. Research has consistently identified that the provision of health care treatment, such as psychological therapy, in itself does not affect work outcomes (Waddell, Burton and Kendall, 2008[42]). What has a proven effect is coordinating employment support with mental health treatment (Lagerveld et al., 2012[43]; Drake and Bond, 2017[44]). For people on sick leave, ensuring health treatments are work-focused is particularly important. Therapy should focus on job-related issues and incorporate job issues early on: the workplace should become one of the foci for improving a person's mental outlook, while employees are encouraged to develop a return-to-work plan. This approach has been found to be more effective than standard cognitive behavioural therapy at supporting a return to work (Cullen et al., 2018[45]). Furthermore, people with mental health conditions who are in work have better outcomes with respect to treatment take-up, duration, and costs than those who are unemployed or inactive (OECD, 2015[1]).

Whilst the New Zealand Health Strategy (Ministry of Health, 2016[15]), and the most recent mental health service development plan, *Rising to the Challenge* (Ministry of Health, 2012[16]) give some recognition to the importance of employment in health care, there is no mention of return to employment as an important outcome and performance measure for health services. There is also an absence of any detail on who is responsible for providing employment support services or how this should be delivered. As a result, the purchasing and provision of employment support is left to the decision of local funders and service providers (Lockett, Waghorn and Kydd, 2018[46]). Consequently, there is a lack of national consistency in supporting people with mental health conditions into employment. There is also a lack of clarity of the roles and responsibilities of the health workforce in relation to supporting people to find work, return to work, and stay in work.

The lack of focus on employment in the health system is further highlighted in the Ministry of Health's *2017 Briefing to the Incoming Minister*. Whilst in this briefing the relationship of employment to health is acknowledged, it is described as a determinant of health "which is outside the health system" (Ministry of Health, 2017[12]). There is also no recognition of the two-way relationship between mental health and work, particularly the impact of a mental health condition on subsequent labour force participation.

Regional health strategies are showing more activity around employment than national policy. Two DHBs have worked together with local non-government organisations to develop *Everyone's Business*, a mental health and employment strategy for the region. The strategy outlines how the region will move to improving the labour force participation of people with mental health conditions, and commitment to implementing the strategy is outlined in the DHBs annual delivery plans. Likewise, the importance of employment for sustained health and wellbeing is recognised in the DHBs five-year strategic plan (Waitemata, 2016[47]). Employment is one of the top three areas for strategic and ground level partnerships. They also propose to measure employment as a marker of improvements in access to mental health treatment.

Employment services integrated with mental health and addiction services aligning with the principles of the Individual Placement and Support evidence-based practices are being delivered in seven DHB regions, and about to commence in two more (Drake and Bond, 2017[44]; Lockett, Waghorn and Kydd, 2018[46]). However, even where IPS is available, access is limited to only some community mental health centres, and not yet linked into specialist mental health services, such as the Māori and Pacific mental health teams and the early intervention in psychosis teams. In other regions, one full-time employment specialist serves the equivalent of three community mental health teams, which produces a diluted service that cannot coordinate effectively employment support with clinical care (Lockett et al., 2018b). IPS services up until recently have been funded through health dollars with two newly established IPS services funded by MSD in 2017 (see Chapter 5).

Like in other countries, IPS programmes in New Zealand have been found to be effective (Porteous and Waghorn, 2007[48]; Browne et al., 2009[49]; Waghorn, Stephenson and Browne, 2011[50]) and to benefit from an integration of services between non-government employment organisations and public mental health and addiction services through the provision of implementation support and technical assistance. Implementation support can include training clinicians on how to have work conversations and to include vocational aspirations as a routine part of assessment and treatment planning. In a recent pilot, the provision of implementation support more than doubled the referrals to employment services, improved fidelity to IPS, increased the reach of the employment services, and strengthened employment outcomes (Te Pou, 2017[51]).

New Zealand also led the development of the *Employment and Mental Health Option Grid*, an evidence-based decision-making tool to help all health practitioners to have work-focused health conversations. However, the uptake and utility of the grid has not been evaluated yet (Reed and Kalaga, 2018[52]).

There have also been a number of pilots to increase the employment focus of primary care but pilots are short-term and small scale. Those working directly in primary care teams are showing promising results (see Chapter 5).

In 2016, RANZCP issued updated clinical guidance on the management of psychosis and schizophrenia. The importance of increasing access to employment services through the inclusion of employment specialists in mental health teams is a key recommendation

(Galletly et al., 2016[53]). In contrast, the BPAC[NZ] management of depression guidance does not mention employment at all. The most recent RANZCP guidance on the management of mood disorders has one mention of employment and housing in the management of major depressive disorder (Malhi et al., 2015), but does not include any of the evidence on the efficacy of employment support integrated in mental health services.

Anecdotal accounts of primary care's understanding and utilisation of the links between health and employment services in relation to injury are prevalent through their experience of working with ACC. ACC provides a range of supports to primary care including treatment and vocational rehabilitation services for patients with ACC claims, as well as online and telephone advice for health practitioners. One ACC vocational rehabilitation service includes *Stay at Work* which take a team-based approach working with the person, their whānau, the GP and other health practitioners, the employer, and a rehabilitation provider. This approach should be extended to people with mental health conditions and the understanding of the interrelationship between health and work that it has no doubt stimulated in primary care, can then be utilised for mental health as well as injury.

New Zealand needs to build a comprehensive programme of national access to integrated psychological therapies and employment support. This could offer different approaches, for example e-therapy with employment support. Programme design and delivery needs to be led by the communities to which they are targeted.

Conclusion

In 1999, the Mental Health Commission published a discussion paper on issues and opportunities in employment and mental health, in order to improve the employment responses for people who experience mental health conditions and addiction (Mental Health Commission, 1999[54]). This paper called for an "integrated public policy response" across mental health, labour market and income support policies and highlighted the lack of information on the "needs, numbers and trends" of people with mental health conditions seeking employment and the lacking "coordination between mental health and employment services". It also concluded that "there appears to be no overarching policy framework and responsibilities are split between a number of Government agencies".

Nineteen years on, the situation appears not to have changed enough. Much of the lack of change is likely to be explained by the complexity and fragmentation of the health system, coupled with an underinvestment in mental health services and primary care services over many years. However, work is underway to strengthen the models of care in primary care to respond more effectively to people presenting with mental health conditions, and to increase access to psychological therapy and employment support.

New Zealand's sustained national awareness and anti-discrimination programmes, which are now focusing on health care settings and workplaces, offer a good platform from which to strengthen the employment focus of mental health care.

Whilst mental health care remains strongly focused on specialist services and reliant on pharmacological treatments this will severely limit the system's ability to support job retention, increase return-to-work rates, and improve labour force participation more generally for people with mental health conditions.

Greater access to psychological treatments, including e-therapies is developed. The scale up of these programmes provides a good opportunity to integrate them with employment support services and to strengthen the links between mental health care and work.

Primary and community health practitioners are innovating new models of care, and culturally informed programmes and support services. As these are grown, and the mental health capacity of primary care strengthened, this is the ideal time to build in training and guidelines around mental health and work, particularly around managing sickness absence and supporting return to or take up, of work.

The presence of ACC has developed and strengthened the employment focus of the health insurance system for injury, but it has also created a two-tier health system where access to treatment and vocational rehabilitation is prioritised for injury and not for illness.

Notes

[1] Strictly speaking, these figures only include spending on general practice. Spending on such items as ambulance services, pharmacies and pharmaceuticals are not included, neither in the data for New Zealand nor in those for other countries. In New Zealand, spending on those items and services exceeds the direct costs for general practice, totalling to around NZD 1.5 billion.

[2] Defined as appointment with secondary or primary care services, where the presenting issues were mental health-related.

[3] Bpac^{nz} is an independent, not for profit organisation advocating for best practice in healthcare treatments and providing education and continuing professional development programmes to health practitioners and health groups across New Zealand.

[4] Pharmac is a Crown Agent. The government allocates a budget each year to Pharmac. Pharmac is responsible for making decisions about which pharmaceuticals and medical equipment to fund. Decisions consider a number of factors, including health needs, the needs of Maori and Pacific peoples, etc., to optimise impact whilst remaining in budget. Pharmac is responsible to the Minister of Health; the Minister cannot override its drug purchase decisions without an Act of Parliament (Productivity Commission, 2015).

References

Allan, K. (2018), *New Zealand's mental health and addiction services – The monitoring and advocacy report of the Mental Health Commissioner*, Office of the Health and Disability Commissioner, Wellington, https://www.hdc.org.nz/media/4688/mental-health-commissioners-monitoring-and-advocacy-report-2018.pdf (accessed on 28 October 2018). [10]

Bassilios, B. et al. (2013), *Evaluating the Access to Allied Psychological Services (ATAPS) component of the Better Outcomes in Mental Health Care (BOiMHC) program: Ten year consolidated ATAPS evaluation report*, Centre for Mental Health, The University of Melbourne, https://www.researchgate.net/publication/275518921_Evaluating_the_Access_to_Allied_Psychological_Services_ATAPS_component_of_the_Better_Outcomes_in_Mental_Health_Care_BOiMHC_program_Ten_year_consolidated_ATAPS_evaluation_report (accessed on 28 October 2018). [34]

bpac (2017), *The role of medicines in the management of depression in primary care*, bpac better medicine, Dunedin, http://www.bpac.org.nz (accessed on 28 October 2018). [32]

Browne, D. et al. (2009), "Developing high performing employment services for people with mental illness", *International Journal of Therapy and Rehabilitation*, Vol. 16/9, pp. 502-511, http://dx.doi.org/10.12968/ijtr.2009.16.9.43769. [49]

Cullen, K. et al. (2018), "Effectiveness of Workplace Interventions in Return-to-Work for Musculoskeletal, Pain-Related and Mental Health Conditions: An Update of the Evidence and Messages for Practitioners", *Journal of Occupational Rehabilitation*, Vol. 28/1, pp. 1-15, http://dx.doi.org/10.1007/s10926-016-9690-x. [45]

Cunningham, R., D. Peterson and S. Collings (2017), "Like Minds, Like Mine: Seventeen Years of Countering Stigma and Discrimination Against People with Experience of Mental Distress in New Zealand", in *The Stigma of Mental Illness - End of the Story?*, Springer International Publishing, Cham, http://dx.doi.org/10.1007/978-3-319-27839-1_15. [3]

Dowell, A. et al. (2009), *Evaluation of the Primary Mental Health Initiatives: Summary Report 2008*, University of Otago and Ministry of Health, Wellington, http://www.moh.govt.nz (accessed on 28 October 2018). [38]

Downs, A. (2017), *From Theory to Practice: The Promise of Primary Care in New Zealand*, Fulbright New Zealand, Wellington, http://www.fulbright.org.nz (accessed on 28 October 2018). [9]

Drake, R. and G. Bond (2017), "Individual Placement and Support: Penetration and New Populations", *Administration and Policy in Mental Health and Mental Health Services Research*, Vol. 44/3, pp. 309-310, http://dx.doi.org/10.1007/s10488-017-0803-4. [44]

Durie, M. (1997), "Maori Cultural Identity and Its Implications for Mental Health Services", *International Journal of Mental Health*, Vol. 26/3, pp. 23-25, http://dx.doi.org/10.1080/00207411.1997.11449407. [23]

Durie, M. (1984), "Te taha hinengaro: An integrated approach to mental health", *Community Mental Health in New Zealand*, Vol. 1/1, pp. 4-11, http://psycnet.apa.org/record/1986-10014-001 (accessed on 28 October 2018). [25]

Elliot, M. (2016), *People's Mental Health Report*, ActionStation Aotearoa, Wellington, https://static1.squarespace.com/static/58f48f2459cc680bc7a237aa/t/58f5d384b8a79b4768cb93a8/1492505610169/PMHR+%28FINAL%29.pdf (accessed on 28 October 2018). [24]

Galletly, C. et al. (2016), "Royal Australian and New Zealand College of Psychiatrists clinical practice guidelines for the management of schizophrenia and related disorders", *Australian & New Zealand Journal of Psychiatry*, Vol. 50/5, pp. 410-472, http://dx.doi.org/10.1177/0004867416641195. [53]

Koning, P. (2004), "Estimating the impact of experience rating on the inflow into disability insurance in the Netherlands", *CPB Discussion Paper*, https://ideas.repec.org/p/cpb/discus/37.html (accessed on 22 October 2018). [41]

KPMG (2013), *Value for Money Review of the National Depression Initiative Programme*, Ministry of Health, Wellington, https://www.health.govt.nz/publication/value-money-review-national-depression-initiative-programme (accessed on 28 October 2018). [35]

Kvalsvig, A. (2018), *Wellbeing and Mental Distress in Aotearoa New Zealand: Snapshot 2016*, Health Promotion Agency, Wellington, http://www.hpa.org.nz (accessed on 28 October 2018). [6]

Lagerveld, S. et al. (2012), "Work-focused treatment of common mental disorders and return to work: A comparative outcome study.", *Journal of Occupational Health Psychology*, Vol. 17/2, pp. 220-234, http://dx.doi.org/10.1037/a0027049. [43]

Lockett, H. et al. (2018), "Primary healthcare utilisation among adults with mood and anxiety disorders: an analysis of the New Zealand Health Survey", *Journal of Primary Health Care*, Vol. 10/1, p. 68, http://dx.doi.org/10.1071/HC17077. [27]

Lockett, H., G. Waghorn and R. Kydd (2018), "Policy barriers to evidence-based practices in vocational rehabilitation for people with psychiatric disabilities in New Zealand", *Work*, Vol. 60/3, pp. 421-435, http://dx.doi.org/10.3233/WOR-182752. [46]

MaGPIe Research Group (2003), "The nature and prevalence of psychological problems in New Zealand primary healthcare: a report on Mental Health and General Practice Investigation (MaGPIe).", *The New Zealand medical journal*, Vol. 116/1171, p. U379, http://www.ncbi.nlm.nih.gov/pubmed/12740629 (accessed on 28 October 2018). [37]

Malatest (2017), *Impact Evaluation of MH101*, Malatest International, Wellington, http://malatest-intl.com/ (accessed on 28 October 2018). [7]

Mental Health Commission (2012), *Blueprint II: Improving mental health and wellbeing for all New Zealand: How things need to be*, Mental Health Commission New Zealand, Wellington, http://www.hdc.org.nz (accessed on 28 October 2018). [17]

Mental Health Commission (1999), *Employment And Mental Health Issues And Opportunities A Discussion Paper*, Mental Health Commission New Zealand, Wellington, http://www.mhc.govt.nz (accessed on 28 October 2018). [54]

Merry, S. et al. (2012), "The effectiveness of SPARX, a computerised self help intervention for adolescents seeking help for depression: randomised controlled non-inferiority trial.", *BMJ (Clinical research ed.)*, Vol. 344, p. e2598, http://dx.doi.org/10.1136/BMJ.E2598. [36]

Ministry of Health (2018), *Mental Health and Addiction Workforce Action Plan 2017–2021*, Ministry of Health, Wellington, https://www.health.govt.nz/system/files/documents/publications/mental-health-addiction-workforce-action-plan-2017-2021-2nd-edn-apr18.pdf (accessed on 28 October 2018). [29]

Ministry of Health (2017), *Briefing to the Incoming Minister of Health: The New Zealand Health and Disability System*, Ministry of Health, Wellington, https://www.health.govt.nz/system/files/documents/publications/briefing-to-the-incoming-minister-of-health-2017-the-new-zealand-health-and-disability-system_0.pdf (accessed on 28 October 2018). [12]

Ministry of Health (2017), *Office of the Director of Mental Health Annual Report 2016*, Ministry of Health, Wellington, https://www.health.govt.nz/system/files/documents/publications/office-of-the-director-of-mental-health-annual-report-2016-dec17-v2.pdf (accessed on 28 October 2018). [21]

Ministry of Health (2016), *New Zealand Health Strategy 2016*, Ministry of Health, Wellington, https://www.health.govt.nz/publication/new-zealand-health-strategy-2016 (accessed on 28 October 2018). [15]

Ministry of Health (2014), *Strengthening He Korowai Oranga*, Ministry of Health, Wellington, https://www.health.govt.nz/our-work/populations/maori-health/he-korowai-oranga/strengthening-he-korowai-oranga (accessed on 28 October 2018). [19]

Ministry of Health (2012), *Rising to the Challenge: The Mental Health and Addiction Service Development Plan 2012-2017*, Ministry of Health, Wellington, http://www.health.govt.nz (accessed on 28 October 2018). [16]

New Zealand Treasury (2018), *Financial Statements of the Government of New Zealand*, New Zealand Treasury, Wellington, https://treasury.govt.nz/publications/year-end/financial-statements-2018 (accessed on 28 October 2018). [11]

NZQA (2017), *Report of External Evaluation and Review: Blueprint NZ Limited*, New Zealand Qualifications Authority, Wellington, http://www.nzqa.govt.nz/providers/nqf- (accessed on 28 October 2018). [8]

OAG (2013), *Regional services planning in the health sector*, Office of the Auditor-General, Wellington, http://www.oag.govt.nz (accessed on 28 October 2018). [31]

Oakley Browne, M. et al. (2006), *Te Rau Hinengaro – The New Zealand Mental Health Survey: Summary*, Ministry of Health, Wellington, https://www.health.govt.nz/system/files/documents/publications/mental-health-survey-summary.pdf (accessed on 28 October 2018). [20]

OECD (2015), *Fit Mind, Fit Job: From evidence to practice in mental health and work.*, OECD Publishing, Paris. [1]

OECD (2015), *Mental Health and Work: Australia*, Mental Health and Work, OECD Publishing, Paris, http://dx.doi.org/10.1787/9789264246591-en. [13]

OECD (2014), *Mental Health and Work: Netherlands*, Mental Health and Work, OECD Publishing, Paris, http://dx.doi.org/10.1787/9789264223301-en. [39]

Pitama, S. et al. (2007), "Meihana Model: A Clinical Assessment Framework", *New Zealand Journal of Psychology*, Vol. 36/3, http://www.psychology.org.nz/wp-content/uploads/Pitamaetal_NZJP36-3_pg118.pdf (accessed on 28 October 2018). [22]

Platform Trust & Te Pou (2015), *On Track: Knowing where we are going*, Te Pou o Te Whakaaro Nui, Auckland, https://www.tepou.co.nz/uploads/files/resource-assets/on-track-knowing-where-we-are-going.pdf (accessed on 28 October 2018). [14]

Porteous, N. and G. Waghorn (2007), "Implementing Evidence-Based Employment Services in New Zealand for Young Adults with Psychosis: Progress during the First Five Years", *British Journal of Occupational Therapy*, Vol. 70/12, pp. 521-526, http://dx.doi.org/10.1177/030802260707001204. [48]

Potter, J. et al. (2017), *Toward a Whole of Government/Whole of Nation Approach to Mental Health*, Office of the prime minister's chief science advisor, Wellington, http://www.pmcsa.org.nz/wp-content/uploads/17-07- (accessed on 28 October 2018). [28]

Productivity Commission (2015), *More effective social services*, New Zealand Productivity Commission, Wellington, https://www.productivity.govt.nz/sites/default/files/social-services-final-report-summary-version.pdf (accessed on 28 October 2018). [26]

Reed, K. and H. Kalaga (2018), "Focusing on employment in primary mental health care: A scoping review", *Work*, Vol. 59/1, pp. 3-13, http://dx.doi.org/10.3233/WOR-172665. [52]

Te Pou (2017), *Getting the right people and skills in the future workforce: Workforce planning guide*, Te Pou o te Whakaaro Nui, Auckland, http://www.tepou.co.nz. (accessed on 28 October 2018). [40]

Te Pou (2017), *IPS implementation manager evaluation: Final report*, Te Pou o te Whakaaro Nui, Auckland, https://www.tepou.co.nz/uploads/files/FINAL%20outcomes%20report%20IPS%20Implementation%20manager.pdf (accessed on 28 October 2018). [51]

Te Pou (2014), *The physical health of people with a serious mental illness and/or addiction: An evidence review*, Te Pou o te Whakaaro Nui, Auckland, http://www.tepou.co.nz (accessed on 28 October 2018). [30]

Te Pou (2012), *Talking Therapies: Where to next?*, Te Pou o te Whakaaro Nui, Auckland, http://www.tepou.co.nz (accessed on 28 October 2018). [33]

Thornicroft, C. et al. (2014), "Impact of the "Like Minds, Like Mine" anti-stigma and discrimination campaign in New Zealand on anticipated and experienced discrimination", *Australian & New Zealand Journal of Psychiatry*, Vol. 48/4, pp. 360-370, http://dx.doi.org/10.1177/0004867413512687. [5]

Thornicroft, G. et al. (2016), "Evidence for effective interventions to reduce mental-health-related stigma and discrimination.", *The Lancet (London, England)*, Vol. 387/10023, pp. 1123-1132, http://dx.doi.org/10.1016/S0140-6736(15)00298-6. [2]

Waddell, G., K. Burton and N. Kendall (2008), *VOCATIONAL REHABILITATION: WHAT WORKS, FOR WHOM, AND WHEN?*, The Stationary Office, London, http://www.tso.co.uk (accessed on 28 October 2018). [42]

Waghorn, G., A. Stephenson and D. Browne (2011), "The Importance of Service Integration in Developing Effective Employment Services for People with Severe Mental Health Conditions", *British Journal of Occupational Therapy*, Vol. 74/7, pp. 339-347, http://dx.doi.org/10.4276/030802211X13099513661153. [50]

Waitemata (2016), *Our health in mind: A five-year strategic plan 2016-2021*, Waitemata District Health Board, Auckland, http://www.waitematadhb.govt.nz/assets/Documents/action-plans/OurHealthInMind.pdf (accessed on 28 October 2018). [47]

Workforce Service Review Working Group (2011), *Towards the Next Wave of Mental Health and Addiction Services and Capability*, Ministry of Health, Wellington, https://www.health.govt.nz/system/files/documents/pages/mental-health-workforce-service-review.pdf (accessed on 28 October 2018). [18]

Wyllie, A. and J. Lauder (2012), *IMPACTS OF NATIONAL MEDIA CAMPAIGN TO COUNTER STIGMA AND DISCRIMINATION ASSOCIATED WITH MENTAL ILLNESS*, Phoenix Research and Ministry of Health, Wellington, http://www.likeminds.org.nz/assets/Uploads/Impacts-of-national-media.pdf (accessed on 28 October 2018). [4]

Chapter 3. Mental resilience and labour market transitions of youth in New Zealand

This chapter evaluates policies and programmes aimed at promoting the mental health of New Zealand's children and youth. The analysis looks at five questions in particular: How does New Zealand's education system promote mental wellbeing and psychological resilience? In what ways do schools intervene when warning signs emerge? What mental health services may young people access through the health care and community system? How do schools and universities stem disengagement and attrition from the education system? What policies and programmes are in place to help vulnerable young people transition into further education or into employment? The analysis uses the OECD's (2015) Council Recommendation on Integrated Mental Health, Skills and Work Policy *as the primary benchmark for best practices in this field.*

Introduction

Policy aimed at investing in a mentally healthy workforce needs to include a focus on the young generation given that 50% of all mental health conditions start before the age of 14 (OECD, 2015[1]). The formative years are a critical time to stimulate self-understanding, emotional maturity and psychological resilience. The ability of primary, secondary and tertiary education institutions to ensure mental wellbeing among their students factors strongly into countries' capabilities around skills development and, ultimately, the fulfilment of economic potential. As the average time to first treatment of mental health conditions runs up to 12 years after onset, children and adolescents are unlikely to get into contact with mental health services unless the impact of the condition becomes serious. The education system has an important role in providing early support for those who show signs of mental health conditions at an early age.

Good educational attainment is essential for a successful transition into the labour market, but children and adolescents who experience mental ill-health are less likely to engage fully in school; less likely to achieve well in their qualifications; and consequently less likely to progress into a fulfilling career. School policies are needed that focus on supporting this group. Not only for young people with severe mental health conditions, for whom some policy is often in place, but especially so for the majority of young people with mild and moderate mental health problems who often are not eligible for specialised health, social and educational support.

Research has shown that youth in New Zealand often struggle with mental health issues. According to the *Youth 2000 Study*, surveying 10 000 secondary school pupils from across New Zealand , 16% of boys and 9% of girls reported clinically significant symptoms of depression; 8% and 29%, respectively, admitted deliberate self-harm in the past 12 months; 10% and 21% serious thoughts about suicide; and 2% and 6% suicide attempts (Clark et al., 2013[2]). The suicide rate for 15-19 year old New Zealand ers in 2013 was 18 per 100 000 compared to 7.4 per 100 000 on average for all OECD countries (OECD, 2017[3]). This accounted for 35% of all deaths in this age group. Like many other social and health outcomes, suicide rates in New Zealand vary starkly by ethnic group: Māori males aged 15-19 years are almost three times more likely to commit suicide than their peers of European ethnicity and Māori females even six times, with suicide rates generally being significantly higher among males than females (Ministry of Health, 2016[4]).

Research has also shown a strong link between child and youth mental health and poverty, concluding that a mental health strategy for children should sit alongside a comprehensive programme to alleviate poverty (Gibson et al., 2017[5]). This is an important aspect but going beyond the remit of this chapter. Increased resources in low-income can reduce anxiety, stress and depression, irrespective of age (Cooper and Stewart, 2015[6]).

The main challenges for youth and education policies

The OECD *Recommendation of the Council on Integrated Mental Health, Skills and Work Policy* calls upon its member countries to: "seek to improve educational outcomes and transitions into further and higher education and the labour market of young people living with mental health conditions", detailing key priorities for action policy makers should consider (OECD, 2015[7]).

Table 3.1 gives an assessment of New Zealand's performance in each of these policy areas and provides corresponding policy recommendations. In summary:

Table 3.1. New Zealand's performance regarding the OECD Council Recommendations around improving educational outcomes and labour market transitions for young people

	OECD Council Recommendation	New Zealand's performance	Suggested actions
A	Monitor and improve the overall school climate to promote **social-emotional learning, mental health and wellbeing** of all children and youth through whole-of-school-based interventions and the prevention of mental stress and bullying.	Strong focus in schools on positive mental health and resilience and strong well-being commitment in the school curriculum. Strong focus on managing behaviour, e.g. through the Positive Behaviour for Learning (PB4L) initiative. B4 School Check to detect problems early. Additional learning support for vulnerable students through Ongoing Resourcing Scheme and Resource Teachers: Learning & Behaviour.	Ensure every child can benefit from the available support by increasing take-up of PB4L School-Wide, and tailoring services and guidelines to vulnerable schools and groups of students. Increase the attention to mental health and bullying prevention in existing programmes. Use "B4 School Check" to identify emotional issues or barriers.
B	**Improve awareness among education professionals and the families of students**, of mental health conditions young people may experience and the ability to identify problems, while ensuring an adequate number of qualified professionals is available to all educational institutions.	Wide range of mental health training packages and guidance materials for both schools and families; the reach and impact of this training however is unclear. Significant focus on school-based health services, including nurses and counsellors. Youth Mental Health Project introduced and expanded various assessment tools (e.g. HEADS screening tool) and initiatives, which are showing good outcomes.	Stimulate the use of training and guidance materials and introduce mental health as mandatory element in the teacher curriculum. Expand funding for school-based health services (minimum service standards; on-site health teams; lower caseloads per counsellor; expansion to primary schools). Use change in funding formula to secure funding for health services.
C	Promote timely access to **co-ordinated, non-stigmatising support for children and youth** with mental health conditions by better linking primary and mental health services and by an easily accessible non-clinical support structure, which provides comprehensive assistance.	Youth Primary Mental Health Services (YPMHS) upscale primary care for early intervention, and reach out to Māori youth. Relatively high use of secondary mental health care among children and youth, but also long waiting times. Strong structure of Youth One Stop Shops (YOSS) with a focus on integrated services for youth aged 10-25 years.	Secure and expand YPMHS funding. Move to stepped-care service model with easy access and referral. Try out integration of primary and secondary youth health services. Secure YOSS funding and expand its counselling capacity. Better integrate YPMHS with YOSS.
D	Invest in the **prevention of early school leaving at all ages** and support for school-leavers living with mental health conditions, with a view to reconnect those students with the education system and labour market.	Large inequality in education outcomes, high attrition from tertiary education, and poor outcomes for the NEET population. Effective support for potential school leavers through the Attendance Service. Various alternative learning pathways.	Ensure that alternative pathways are providing high-quality support. Prioritise support for Māori youth. Better link programmes targeted to potential school leavers with other youth services, such as YOSS, Youthline and YPMHS.
E	Provide **non-stigmatising support for the transition from school** to higher education and work for students with mental health problems through well-integrated services.	Range of initiatives under the Youth Guarantee to widen learning options and improve transition into employment. Youth Service (under Work and Income) targeted at NEETs and beneficiaries.	Expand Youth Guarantee initiatives with good outcomes and secure the same outcomes for Māori youth. Strengthen Youth Service monitoring and evaluation and strengthen the link with education institutions.

Source: Authors' own assessment based on all of the evidence collected in this chapter.

New Zealand'seducation system has a strong focus on positive mental health and well-being and provides considerable resources for i) additional learning support for vulnerable pupils and ii) managing undesirable behaviour. Education outcomes, however, remain highly unequal suggesting that disadvantaged schools and groups of students are not able to benefit sufficiently from the approach taken and the resources provided.

New Zealand offers various mental health trainings to schools and families and is very aware of the need to provide school-based health services and to identify problems early on. In effect, however, not all schools have effective on-site health and mental health services in place, and the available number of health professionals is insufficient. Owing to schools' autonomy, there are no minimum requirements, which all schools would have to follow. National policy should strengthen the availability and consistency of school-based mental health training and services across the country. Resources need allocating according to need and a particular focus on Māori youth.

Use of specialised mental health care is high among New Zealand youth whereas primary mental health services are under-resourced despite recent efforts to up-scale primary care for prevention and early intervention. Youth One Stop shops are an exemplary service, which is easily accessible and provides all-inclusive supports; but resources are insufficient to satisfy the demand and the connection with other services is still insufficient.

New Zealand pays much attention to the prevention of early school leaving, through an effective Attendance Service, and provides a range of alternative learning pathways to help students back into school or complete education. Māori youth are highly over-represented in all these pathways, which, however, produce much poorer outcomes than regular schools, and would benefit from stronger links with other youth services.

New Zealand offers a number of initiatives under its Youth Guarantee that aim to improve the transition into further education and/or employment, predominantly by making the curriculum more relevant, including through vocationally focused and workplace-based learning opportunities. So far, however, these programmes have failed to help more Māori youth into employment. Many of them end up in the Youth Service, targeted at NEETs and people in receipt of youth payments but with limited evidence on its effectiveness.

Mental wellbeing in school

New Zealand's education system has a strong commitment to nurturing mental wellbeing and enhancing the resilience of young people. It is ahead of some other OECD countries with concepts of wellbeing and positive mental health built into the curriculum and by having in place strong institutions for detecting and responding to potential signs of behavioural or psychological needs among learners. The evidence gathered suggests New Zealand has set up multiple promising initiatives in this area. The main challenge is to ensure every child and youth can benefit from the strength of the system, irrespective of social background, location and ethnicity, which in turn requires adequate tailoring to vulnerable schools and groups of students.

Wellbeing is in the curriculum but some schools struggle with implementation

Laws in New Zealand mandate schools to ensure pupils' wellbeing. This includes a focus on students' satisfaction with life at school, their engagement with learning and their social-emotional behaviour. Student wellbeing is defined as a sustainable state, characterised by predominantly positive feelings and attitude, positive relationships at school, resilience, self-optimism and a high level of satisfaction with learning experiences (Education Review Office, 2013[8]). New Zealand's Education Council maintains a strict professional code and key criteria for registered school teachers, formally committing them to promoting pupils' wellbeing on five key fronts: physical, emotional, social, intellectual and spiritual. A set of *National Administration Guidelines* formally mandate schools' management boards to maintain safe physical and emotional environments.

Above all, mental wellbeing, socio-emotional development and psychological resilience are mainstreamed nationally through New Zealand's school curriculum. The primary and secondary curriculum adopts an explicit focus on five "key competencies" all pupils are expected to develop during their compulsory education: *thinking*; *using language, symbols and texts*; *managing self*; *relating to others*; and *participating and contributing* (Ministry of Education, 2017[9]). Tertiary education providers likewise adopt a parallel set of key competencies around *thinking*; *using tools interactively*; *acting autonomously*; and *operating in social groups* (Hipkins, 2006[10]).[1] Nurturing these key competencies is both a means towards improving learning outcomes and a valuable end in itself (Ministry of Education, 2007[11]). Ultimately, the key competencies also ensure a clear focus is maintained within the education system on positive mental health and a clearer understanding of emotions and cognition.[2]

New Zealand's coherent policies and practices in this area are borne out in the available data on school teachers' and families' perceptions around children's wellbeing at school. In a national survey carried out in 2016 by the New Zealand Council for Educational Research (NZCER), the large majority of the surveyed teachers felt their school effectively supported pupils' wellbeing and sense of belonging (85%) and taught emotional skills assertively (86%). Surveyed family members felt equally positively that the school environment promoted wellbeing, a sense of belonging and psychological resilience, with only 2-3% disagreeing on these points (Boyd, Bonne and Berg, 2017[12]).

In 2012, the Education Review Office (ERO) carried out an evaluation of wellbeing practices in primary and lower-secondary schools.[3] ERO's findings categorised the schools into five broad categories (Education Review Office, 2015[13]):

- 11% managed to promote an "extensive focus on student wellbeing" throughout all their activities
- 18% promoted wellbeing well within their own curriculum and response systems
- 48% promoted wellbeing only reasonably well, predominantly relying on a positive atmosphere and respectful relationships to achieve good outcomes
- 20% made rather limited use of wellbeing promotion techniques, focusing predominantly on managing bad behaviour
- 3% were "overwhelmed by wellbeing issues", with few concrete activities manifesting in high staff turnover, low capacity for improvement, unclear values, weak trust and a deep-set dependence on outside support.

Thus, despite the strong focus on pupils' wellbeing in the national curriculum, only 28% of all schools managed to perform satisfactorily and almost a quarter (23%) was unable to integrate wellbeing in their curriculum. Although ERO has developed more detailed guidelines for schools to improve their performance along the desired lines and to engage in effective self-evaluation (Education Review Office, 2016[14]), it would be important to profile the schools struggling with integrating wellbeing initiatives. For example, it would be relevant to know whether schools in more remote areas (potentially having more difficulty with attracting extra services focusing on wellbeing) or with more students with socio-economic disadvantages who face a high risk of developing mental health and social problems belong to the 23% performing poorly. ERO could use such information to tailor guidelines to the challenges that schools performing poorly specifically face.

A focus on managing behaviour but limited attention on preventing bullying

Misbehaviour in school is a significant detriment to learning environments. Behaviours like bullying (including cyber-bullying) can also directly affect pupils' mental wellbeing and feelings of belonging and security. The relative success or failure schools encounter in managing pupils' behaviour can therefore have a significant impact on pupils' overall wellbeing and learning outcomes.

The Ministry of Education undertakes a range of activities to help schools better manage behaviour. Since 2009, its efforts have converged under the Positive Behaviour for Learning (PB4L) initiative. The initiative's flagship scheme is *PB4L School-Wide* – a structured framework to help schools understand and shape the ways in which their environments, rules and practices influence pupils' behavioural choices.

New Zealand's government formally evaluated PB4L School-Wide in 2015. The analysis found that schools using the framework issued fewer formal punishments (like school stand-downs, suspensions, exclusions or expulsions) to pupils; experienced less disruption in class; and reported increases in pupils' concentration and engagement. However, programme uptake is still low, with only 780 schools – roughly one in three schools across New Zealand – currently applying PB4L School-Wide.

The Ministry of Education also provides a range of specific interventions for schools to draw upon in particularly challenging cases. Behaviour Services and Support, for example, provides a local pool of specialists who can work with school-aged children alongside their teachers and family members in cases of extreme behavioural difficulties. Schools may engage such specialists to work with pupils alongside their families, school staff and external specialists to tailor an individualised learning support plan.

Failing all of these interventions, schools are also empowered to issue formal disciplinary measures or, in the worst case, remove a pupil under particularly disruptive circumstances.[4] The Ministry of Education closely monitors such outcomes and responds to requests for support. Administrative data show that the incidence of suspensions decreased by around 50% between 2000 and 2016, from an age-standardised rate of 7.4 suspensions per 1 000 pupils per year to just 3.6 (Ministry of Education, 2018$_{[15]}$). The number of exclusions and expulsions has declined at a similar rate, suggesting that support measures available for schools and students in difficulties have been successful in keeping more students in class and in school. Stand-downs, the lowest degree of a formal disciplinary measure, declined from 24.4 to 20.6 per 1 000 pupils per year over the same period. All disciplinary measures affect Pasifika youth somewhat more often and Māori youth much more often than students from other ethnicities. However, the rate of decline was also largest among Māori youth, resulting in some convergence in outcomes and suggesting that available measures have started to reduce ethnic inequalities.[5]

Specific attention for mental health and for the prevention of bullying seems to be missing in these programmes and interventions. They are geared towards stimulating adequate classroom behaviour among pupils, but bullying is often more covert and conducted outside classrooms. This is worrisome given that the most recent data from the OECD's PISA study reveal high levels of bullying in New Zealand's schools. In 2015, 26% of pupils reported experiencing at least one of the six bullying behaviours a few times a month – the second-highest share among all OECD countries and significantly above the OECD average of below 19% (OECD, 2017$_{[16]}$).

There are a number of initiatives aimed at preventing bullying behaviour, but these are not sufficiently supported by a clear policy on bullying for schools coming from the

Ministry of Education. For example, the Mental Health Foundation organises the annual *Pink Shirt Day* since 2009, delivering coordinated activities in schools and workplaces to end bullying and celebrate diversity. Other initiatives focusing on bullying prevention in schools are organised by KiVa New Zealand and Bullying-free NZ.

Potentially more promising could be the PB4L Restorative Practice initiative, which provides a framework to help schools foster positive relationships, based on values of fairness, dignity, *mana* and universal potential. This includes a focus on relational and problem-solving skills among pupils, which may affect bullying behaviour. However, uptake of PB4L Restorative Practice is even lower than PB4L School-Wide; currently only around 180 schools across New Zealand use the programme. A formal evaluation of PB4L Restorative Practice is underway. It would be advisable to also regularly measure (changes in) bullying behaviour among pupils.[6]

Additional learning support for vulnerable students

New Zealand has highly robust institutions in place for identifying developmental or behavioural difficulties early on and, in turn, providing additional learning support.

New Zealand's Ministry of Health undertakes a mandatory *B4 School Check* (read as: before-school check) to examine the physical, behavioural, social and developmental condition of children aged four. Such checks are performed by nurses through local primary health organisations (PHOs) funded by the district health boards (DHBs). Screening for behavioural and psychological needs consists primarily of the Strengths and Difficulties Questionnaire and the Parental Evaluation of Developmental Status tool. The B4 School Check which reaches some 80% of all New Zealand pre-schoolers provides a valuable benchmark for families and an early warning for potential learning difficulties or special educational needs. The psychological and emotional component of this tool could be expanded to ensure low-threshold psychological support can be delivered early on.

Primary and secondary schools are equipped to cater for a majority of difficulties children encounter around learning, communication and behaviour. Schools can access several types of funding for pupils with moderate or more severe learning or behavioural needs. Pupils with moderate learning or behavioural needs can gain support from local *Resource Teachers: Learning and Behaviour* (RTLB) services, funded by the Ministry of Education. In total, in the school year 2017/2018 almost 1 000 RTLB teachers were available serving approximately 15 350 students, meaning that every resource teacher on average had to support some 16 students, but with considerable regional variation.

Funding for children with more significant educational needs (1-2% of all school pupils) is provided by the Ministry of Education via the *Ongoing Resourcing Scheme* (ORS) (Ministry of Education, 2017[9]). The ORS provides special financial support for pupils with significant learning difficulties to remain among peers within a mainstream education setting. ORS support can be used to engage special teaching staff to deliver one-to-one support in classrooms alongside specialist support for counselling, speech and language therapies and occupational therapy. There is also a choice for some children following an ORS assessment to attend one of currently 30 special schools although the government is aiming to close these schools (Ministry of Education, 2018[15]).

Limited information is available about the extent to which these additional funds and forms of support also reach youth with mental health conditions. Youths with more internalising problems (e.g. anxiety and depressed mood) as opposed to more visible problems (such as disruptive or aggressive behaviour), are especially likely to miss out on additional learning support. Monitoring the share of pupils accessing these schemes by cause and type of problem could provide valuable insight.

Mental health awareness and abilities to intervene early

Improving mental health literacy within school communities and children's homes is a critical lever for positive impacts further down the line. Schools in many OECD countries may fail to recognise or act upon early warning signs of mental distress (OECD, 2015[1]). Specialist staff may be unavailable while ordinary teachers often face time constraints in their day-to-day work or lack the necessary knowledge to deal with such issues. Family members and others may likewise be ill prepared to identify and act upon early signs of mental health issues among youth. Stigma towards mental health conditions often further exacerbates the problems and limits the solutions among schools, homes and communities that fail to address it concertedly.

Awareness-raising and training initiatives need broader implementation

New Zealand has a variety of awareness-raising and training initiatives to improve knowledge around mental health issues affecting children and youth. Some focus more on teachers and school leaders while others target parents, carers and *whanau*.

Schools in New Zealand may address a range of common issues around mental health via the guidance protocols provided by the Ministry of Education and bodies like ERO, NZCER and others. These tend to be evidence-based and draw on practices developed in other countries.

Available teacher training packages and guidance materials that can contribute to improving the situation of youth with mental health conditions include the following:

- Understanding Behaviour, Responding Safely is a training workshop organised directly by the Ministry of Education to teach school staff specific behavioural management techniques. The training focuses on prevention and de-escalation techniques with a proven effect. It is delivered to schools' entire staff alongside ongoing support from local Ministry of Education offices.
- Wellbeing@School is a website supported by the Ministry of Education that allows teachers and school principals to review their own performance around pupils' wellbeing and inclusion. The site hosts a periodic self-assessment tool for individuals and school communities, designed by NZCER. Some 1 200 schools are currently registered to access the site's materials.
- Pause, Breathe, Smile is a training programme organised by the Mental Health Foundation for teachers to deliver mindfulness meditation techniques to children in school. The programme's courses for teachers have currently reached around 200 schools throughout New Zealand . Participation in the programme leads to statistically significant and potentially lasting improvements in children's calmness, attention-keeping, self-awareness, conflict resolution and relationship skills alongside improvements around teachers' wellbeing and job satisfaction (Bernay et al., 2016[17]; Devcich et al., 2017[18]).
- Help for the Tough Times provides advice and guidance for school teachers and principals addressing pupils' mental wellbeing. It is part of the Health Promotion Agency's broader Lowdown youth mental health campaign. Lowdown seeks to help young people talk about and overcome common life issues such as study

stress, sexual identity, isolation, bullying and romantic and peer relationships. The campaign combines social media, digital advertising and street posters with an online forum, self-help materials and useful links.

Beyond supports targeted to classrooms, there are several materials designed in parallel to address children's wellbeing at home and in their local communities. Supports targeted towards parents, guardians and whānau include the following:

- MH101 is a one-day training programme funded by the Ministry of Health to help educate the general population to understand and respond to mental distress or mental health conditions in others. In 2012, modules of MH101 were specifically adapted for meeting young people's needs under the government's Youth Mental Health Project. MH101 is routinely rolled out to staff working in New Zealand's Attendance Service, the Work and Income Youth Service, school-based social services and related occupations.
- Guidelines for supporting young people with stress, anxiety and depression is a publication developed in 2015 to help equip families, friends and whānau with the knowledge and skills to support a young person going through mild or moderate mental distress (Ministry of Social Development, 2015[19]).
- The Mental Health Foundation provides a parallel web-, phone- or text-based support and counselling line called Common Ground to help guide parents, whānau and friends in supporting a young person experiencing mental distress.

Despite such a strong and diverse set of instruments in place, there remains some concern that they are failing to reach a wide-enough audience. An NZCER survey from 2016 revealed unmet needs for training and support around mental health, in particular, with only 20% of teachers indicating they could access training around detecting the signs of mental distress and only 34% of principals reporting that their schools were offering such training. Furthermore, 38% of school principals cited an unmet need for external expertise around mental health and 29% of teachers thought the support within their schools was inadequate (Boyd, Bonne and Berg, 2017[12]).

The inadequate implementation of available instruments in schools may be explained by a lack of regulation. New Zealand's devolved education system offers considerable liberty and flexibility around the training and ongoing development incumbent teachers may receive. This implies that while some school administrators may focus their resources on mental health related training, others will invest in other areas. Information is lacking on how many schools are implementing programmes to improve mental health awareness among teachers. Additional measures are necessary to ensure improved mental health literacy of educational professionals nation-wide. For example, including considerable mental health training in the national teacher curriculum would be a way to realise this.

School-based health services need to be extended and monitored

Schools may provide school-based health services. Such primary care services could involve an on-site primary care nurse, a visiting public health nurse, or a DHB nurse. Earlier models included an affiliated social worker, and this model is continued in some schools. Government-funded school-based health services are available in public secondary schools in the bottom three socio-economic deciles[7] (in the current financial year this is expanded to include decile 4 schools) as well as Teen Parent Units and Special Schools.[8] Within school-based health services, there are some concerns about nurse capacity given a ratio of around 750 students per nurse.

School-based counsellors can be part of the broader school-based health services. They may deliver direct talking therapies alongside specialised screening tools. Those tools used under certain circumstances include the *Patient Health Questionnaire* for picking up on general depression; the *Ask Suicide-Screening Questions* for suicide prevention; and the *CRAFFT Screening Tool* and the *Substances and Choices Scale* for potentially harmful behaviours related to substance use (Best Practice Advocacy Centre New Zealand, 2015[20]). However, according to the New Zealand Association of Counsellors (NZAC), the current counsellors-to-students ratio in secondary schools is inadequate with one counsellor being responsible for up to 1 000 students while a more meaningful ratio would be closer to 1:400. Furthermore, school counsellors mostly work in secondary schools, while better continuity of care would be ensured when they also became employed in primary and intermediate schools.

In 2012, the government launched the *Youth Mental Health Project*, primarily targeting the age group 12-19 and including a range of school-based programmes aimed at closing existing service gaps. This project followed the landmark report "Improving the Transition" which focused on ways to improve mental health outcomes for young people transitioning into adulthood (Gluckman, 2011[21]).

The Youth Mental Health Project launched and financed 26 individual initiatives across the Ministry of Education, Ministry of Health, Ministry of Social Development and *Te Puni Kōkiri* (Ministry of Māori Development).[9] Most initiatives are still ongoing.

One of the most lasting of the 26 initiatives delivered has been the roll-out of the HEADS Assessment addressing young people's experiences and feelings around their home environment (H), education and employment, eating and exercise (E), activities and peers (A), drugs and alcohol, depression and suicide (D), and sexual health, safety and personal strengths (S). HEADS assessment is a confidential, loosely structured interview tapping into each of the topic areas; it provides a valuable screening tool for mental distress and potential vulnerabilities around psychological and emotional health. These interviews are also seen to play a useful role in opening young people up to talking about their feelings and address concerns that may come up in the future. However, nation-wide implementation is challenging. An evaluation of school-based health services in 2012 with a random sample of 90 secondary schools across New Zealand found that only one in five schools routinely perform HEADS assessments (Denny S. et al., 2014[22]). With the recent extension to decile 3 and the ongoing extension to decile 4 schools, such assessments or wellness checks will soon be performed in about 40% of all (secondary) schools.

Several of the other 26 initiatives, aimed at creating more supportive schools for pupils' mental wellbeing, have also had a first impact. First, this includes the national rollout of the PB4L School-Wide initiative, mentioned earlier. Second, a cognitive behavioural therapy programme, the My FRIENDS Youth Resilience Programme, was piloted over a two-year period among approximately 14 000 Year-9 students in 26 schools. Third, the Youth Workers in Low-Decile Secondary School (YWiSS) initiative was piloted in 20 schools with a specific focus on youth with mental health issues. Both pilots showed improved self-management among students (e.g. managing own feelings and thinking about the feelings of others) and the YWiSS pilot showed better school results (Superu, 2016[23]; Macdonald et al., 2015[24]).

Another potentially relevant programme is the Social Workers in Schools (SWiS) service, introduced in 1999 but expanded significantly in 2012-13, with additional funding provided through the Youth Mental Health Project. Initially only available in some primary and intermediate schools, SWiS is now available in all around 700 decile 1-3 schools (up from around 300 schools previously); schools with a large share of Māori and Pacific students. The aim of SWiS is to foster school engagement and protect vulnerable children through the provision of group-based programmes as well as individual casework with children and their families and whanau. A 2018 evaluation of the programme found SWiS is acceptable to service users and successfully engages families and whanau. It also identified positive effects for service users in terms of a reduction in school stand-downs and suspensions and police apprehensions but no overall statistically significant effects, which is due to the small size and low intensity of the programme, with a caseload of 400-700 students per social worker (Wilson et al., 2018[25]).[10]

Comprehensive school-based health and social services affect mental health outcomes, but are not yet common practice in New Zealand. The study mentioned above showed that of the 90 surveyed schools, 12% provided only the minimum requirement of first-aid health services, 56% worked with visiting health professionals and only the remaining 32% provided more comprehensive health services in the form of a health professional (mostly a school nurse) on site (20%) or a collaborative health team on site (12%). Furthermore, in schools with a visiting health professional, 0.8 hour of support per week per 100 students was reported on average, while schools with an on-site health professional or health team reported on average, respectively, 4.2 and 4.8 hours of support per week per 100 students. The study also evaluated how school-based health services affect young people's mental health. Pupils in schools with comprehensive health services (i.e. health professionals on site) were significantly less prone to depression; faced a lower risk of suicide; paid less visits to doctors; and (to some extent) reported safer sexual activity. Overall, the results suggest that pupils benefit from high quality school health services consisting of on-site health professionals who are trained in youth health and have sufficient time to work with their pupils (Denny S. et al., 2014[22]).

The implementation of comprehensive school-based mental health teams in Canterbury after the major earthquake has also been positively received although a formal evaluation on improved mental health outcomes has not yet been performed. The school-based mental health teams deliver interventions such as identifying students with mental health issues and supporting referrals to wider services; assisting schools to understand student behaviour by providing or facilitating workshops; and consulting with parents, teachers and pastoral care teams. These teams have been implemented in 102 primary and secondary schools in the Canterbury region (Superu, 2016[23]).[11]

Schools across New Zealand would benefit from such school-based mental health teams. It would be advisable to explore how a system comparable to the Canterbury one could be translated to a national policy for all schools or at least low-decile schools with a more vulnerable student population. The government's plans to change the decile-based school funding system to a new approach based on students' "risk of not achieving" may provide a good opportunity to include mental health as a new indicator, thereby allowing more funding to implement adequate mental health services for schools with a larger share of pupils with mental health conditions.

The high degree of autonomy for schools in New Zealand provides an opportunity to deliver those services most needed for a school's student population, but monitoring is needed to ensure important issues such as mental health are addressed in all schools. A national or regional monitoring system of school-based (mental) health services is lacking and knowledge is thus limited on the number of schools contracting school nurses, social workers, counsellors and youth mental health professionals and on hours of support that is available per school and per student. Minimum health service standards could be set to ensure all schools are apt to the mental health challenge they are facing.

Adequate low-threshold mental health support for children and young people

Countries commonly struggle to ensure that adequate support and treatment for mental health problems reach young people in a timely way (OECD, 2015[1]). Many such problems may go unreported or undetected over extended periods. Even young people with diagnosed mental health problems can encounter low treatment rates, for example due to long waiting times or high thresholds for entering health services. Misinformation and stigma, in turn, may contribute to making things worse.

A stepped-care approach to mental health for youth can help in developing timely, low-threshold and adequate services. These types of models recommend that the first mild-to-moderate signs of mental ill health are intervened upon by easily accessible support structures and primary care services. More specialised services are added when the severity of need and impact increases. This health services model is increasingly used internationally and has shown to be cost-effective (Ho et al., 2016[26]).

Mental health services for youth need alignment with a stepped-care model

The Youth Primary Mental Health Service (YPMHS), one of the 26 initiatives of the Youth Mental Health Project, has been directed at up-scaling primary care services for young people aged 12-19 with mild-to-moderate mental health conditions. It builds upon the existing Primary Mental Health Services (PMHS) that are embedded in primary care, but rarely delivered to youth. YPMHS was started in 2012 and the implementation and results have been evaluated up until 2015 (Malatest International, 2016[27]).

Under YPMHS, NZD 1.3 million were allocated to the District Health Boards (DHBs) over four years (2012/13 to 2015/16) in order to: (1) expand the age range of primary mental health services; (2) adapt existing services for youth; (3) expand existing NGO or community-based initiatives; and (4) develop new initiatives to meet local needs. YPMHS have been able to reach 3 000 to 4 200 youth each quarter, including more females than males (around 60-65% of the recipients were female) and a high share of Māori youth (almost one-third of the clients, compared to 21% of Māori youth in the total youth population). The most frequently used interventions were individual counselling (brief intervention) and packages of care with three to six counselling sessions.

YPMHS funding has been used to develop youth-friendly primary mental health services, but it is unclear whether services are easily accessible for youth and if young people receive the right services. General practices are the main access point for youth primary mental health care. However, the New Zealand Health Survey 2014/15 showed that not all young people go to a general practice: unmet need reaches a level of 22%. To increase access, YPMHS funding may need a stronger focus on entry points outside general practice, such as NGO or community-based initiatives who deliver multiple youth-specific services. In terms of actual services, it is essential that providers under YPMHS are equipped to provide first support to youth with mental health issues and can refer them easily to additional services if needed. The YPMHS evaluation showed that of the 317 surveyed providers (primarily GPs and practice nurses in primary care), as many as 20% were only a little confident in identifying and helping a young person with mental health conditions (Malatest International, 2016[27]). Some 30-50% were only a little or not at all confident in providing certain common interventions such as talking therapies or motivational interviewing. While four in five providers indicated they could refer clients to other services, one in two mentioned a lack of suitable services as a major barrier to providing good care for youth with mental health problems. Accessing specific services showed to be particularly difficult for Māori and Pacific youth, according to more than 70% of the providers. Among the main recommendations from the YPMHS evaluation are to invest in: (1) reducing access barriers for help-seeking youth; (2) increasing the capacity of youth-specific services; and (3) developing the youth workforce.

A well-functioning stepped-care model would include easy referral, when needed, from primary to specialised mental health care. This is not always the case. Almost two in three YPMHS providers indicated that secondary mental health services were not at all or somewhat difficult to access. Around 60% experienced waiting times for such referrals to specialists as a major or substantial barrier to providing care to young people with mental health conditions. Young people aged 0-19 face longer waiting times for mental health and addiction services than adults, with fewer than 70% receiving a first appointment within three weeks of their referral, below the government's target of 80% (Office of the Health and Disability Commissioner, 2018[28]). YPMHS evaluation thus recommended increasing investments in the development of efficient and cohesive youth mental health services including the co-location of primary and specialist youth services.

Although referral to youth specialised mental health services is not without issues, these specialised services more frequently see young people than adults. According to data from the Programme for the Integration of Mental Health Data (PRIMHD), 7% of young people aged 15-19 accessed mental health and addictions services in New Zealand during the 12 months to July 2017. This was a higher rate than for any other age-bracket, with 10-14 year-olds and 20-24 year-olds following with over 5% (Figure 3.1, Panel A). Support was accessed by females and males at similar rates in every age group, except 5-9 year-olds where boys far outnumbered girls (Panel B). The Māori population accessed support at much higher rates than any other ethnic group (Panel C). Socio-economic deprivation also plays an important role in access to mental health and addiction services. Based on a composite index of socio-economic deprivation, those living in the worst-off areas accessed services at significantly higher rates than those in other locations (Panel D).

Today's rates of access to mental health and addiction services among children and youth are a big improvement on the situation from a decade ago. The Mental Health Commission (1998[29]) established national targets for access to public mental health and addiction services under its "Blueprint for mental health services in New Zealand ", which continues to be referenced today. Alongside an overall target of 3% of the population each year, on aggregate, the Blueprint introduced age-disaggregated targets for child and adolescent services to reach 3% of the population aged 0-19 in every six-month period, including: 1.0% among children aged 0-9; 3.9% among adolescents aged 10-14; 5.5% among young people aged 15-19; and 6.0% among the Māori community aged 0-19. Official reports for the year to July 2017 confirm that the current system well exceeds these targets and that the growth in access from children and adolescents exceeds that of the adult population (Office of the Health and Disability Commissioner, 2018[28]).

The rise in access rates to specialised mental health care for young people partly follows the continual increase in funding for child and adolescent mental health and addiction services. However, it may also partly reflect difficulties for some groups of the population, especially young Māori and other disadvantaged groups, in accessing primary care. Primary and specialised care are organised very differently in New Zealand (see Chapter 2); while the latter is free of charge, use of primary care comes with considerable co-payment for the users although children under age 13 (and soon age 14) are free. This could be an incentive to seek care from the specialised sector when in fact the primary care sector could have been the most suitable provider of care, or at least a good first point of call. However, the extent to which such financing constraints may stimulate an under-use of primary care and an over-use of specialised care is unknown.

Figure 3.1. Young people have the highest access to mental health and addiction services of any age group in New Zealand

Rate of clients seen by mental health and addiction services in New Zealand by age group and other variables, 1 July 2016-30 June 2017 (clients seen per 100 000 of the relevant population group)

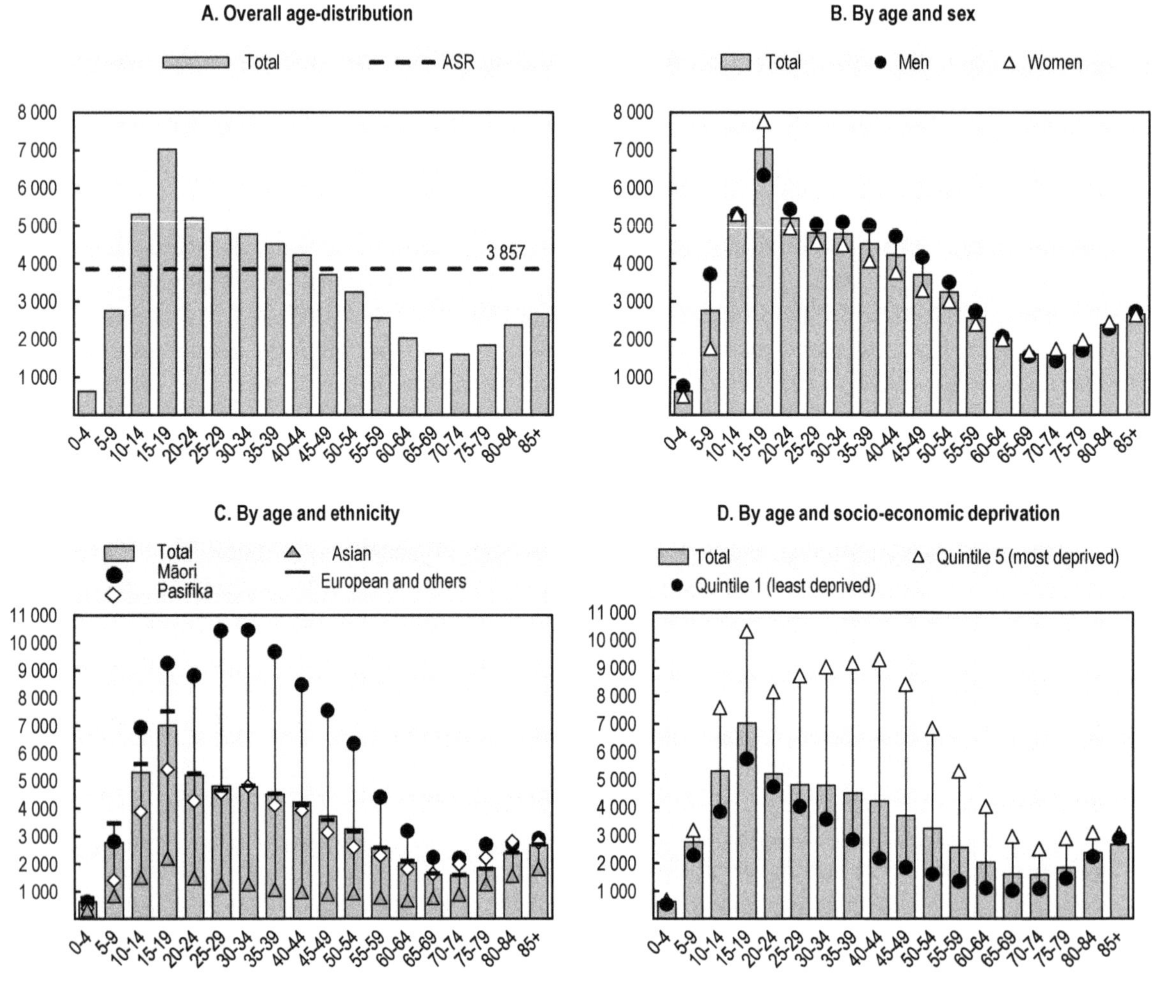

Note: "Clients seen" include users of mental health and addiction services, including remote services (e.g. telephone contact with a clinician). "ASR" indicates the age-standardised rate for the population as a whole. Socio-economic deprivation is for small geographic areas, using variables from the 2006 Census of Populations and Dwellings (full methodology is available from www.health.govt.nz; search for "NZDep2006 Index of Deprivation"). The sum of clients seen across all deprivation quintiles is greater than the total number of clients, as some clients were recorded in more than one quintile during this period.
Source: Programme for the Integration of Mental Health Data (PRIMHD).

StatLink http://dx.doi.org/10.1787//888933845415

Within the specialised sector, community teams (consisting of various mental health professionals) accounted for virtually all mental health care delivered to children during the 12 months to July 2015, including around 93% of the contacts made with 0-4 and 5-9 year-olds (Figure 3.2). Other specialised teams are used more and more frequently among older age groups. Alcohol and drug teams, for example, accounted for 17% of contacts made with 10-14-year-olds, rising to 28% among 25-29 year olds.

Figure 3.2. Community teams in New Zealand are the main provider of specialised mental health services for children

Clients seen by mental health and addiction services in New Zealand by age and team type, 1 July 2014-30 June 2015 (as a percentage of the total contacts by each team)

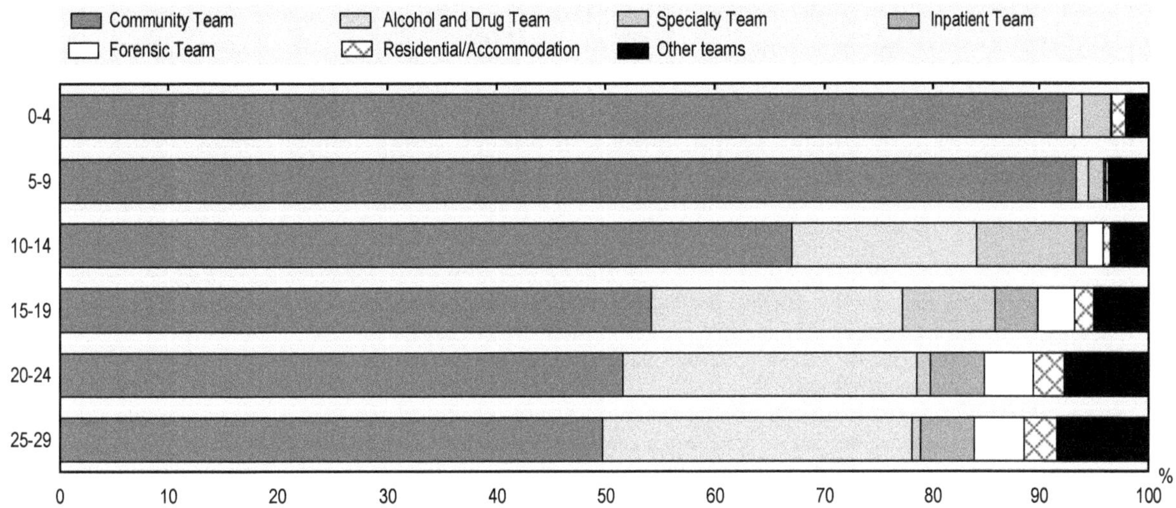

Note: Data represent total contacts per team and may exceed the total number of individual clients within the system due to some double counting (i.e. where a client has had contact with more than one type of team). A small number of teams have been miscoded to inpatient team type, slightly overestimating the inpatient team share. The Ministry of Health is working with the relevant teams to correct this. "Others" include needs assessment and service coordination teams, eating disorder teams, co-existing problems teams, intellectual disability dual-diagnosis teams, specialist psychotherapy teams and early intervention teams.
Source: Programme for the Integration of Mental Health Data (PRIMHD).

StatLink http://dx.doi.org/10.1787/888933845434

In line with a stepped model of care, young people would ideally not only access primary (mental) health services before accessing specialised care but also be referred back to primary care after specialised treatment has finished. This enables a low-threshold and low-cost follow-up of young people ensuring a quick response to recurring problems and good monitoring of treatment compliance. Data on discharge pathways by specialised youth mental health services seem to indicate that this is not common practice in New Zealand, however. More than 50% of child clients, aged 0-9, were discharged without any further referral. This was likewise the case for more than 40% of adolescents and young adults (Figure 3.3), likely being another proof of a certain disconnection in New Zealand between privately run primary care practices and publicly-funded secondary care units.

Figure 3.3. Most children and adolescents in New Zealand are referred to mental health and addiction services by their GPs or their family and most are discharged back home

New referrals to and discharges from mental health and addiction services in New Zealand according to the client's age and the source of referral or destination of discharge, 1 July 2014-30 June 2015

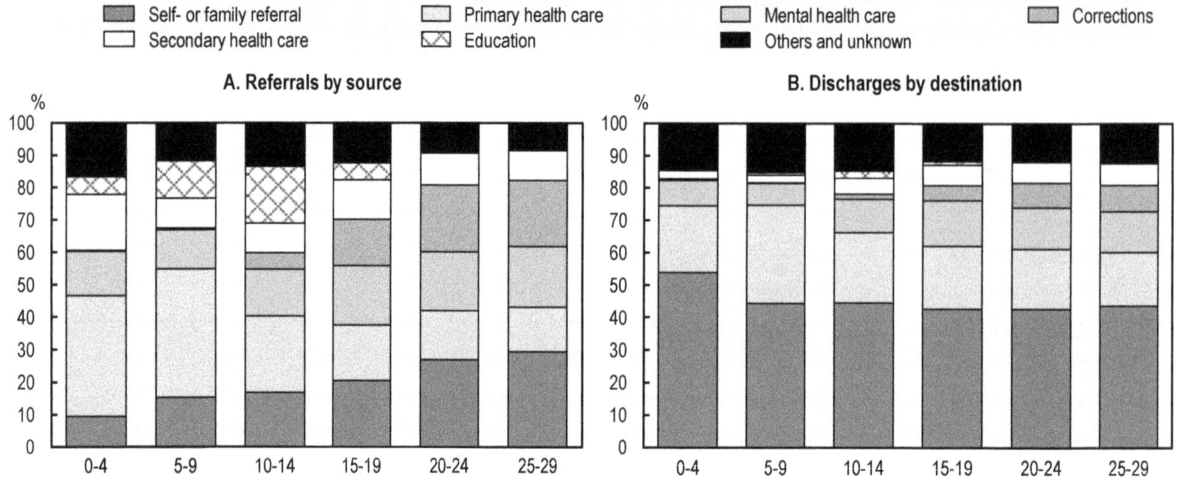

Note: A client can have more than one referral open at one time and might, therefore, be counted against more than one referral source. New referrals are defined as those made within the year to 30 June 2015. The groupings shown are aggregates of multiple categories within the original data:

- *Self- or family referral* includes referrals made by clients themselves, by their relatives or by Māori or Pasifika community groups.
- *Primary health care* referrals and discharges include those made from or to a general practitioner, private practitioner, paediatrics service or a needs assessment and co-ordination service.
- *Mental health care* referrals and discharges include those made from or to an adult community mental health service; a child, adolescent, family or whānau mental health service; a psychiatric inpatient or outpatient service; or a mental health residential service.
- *Corrections* referrals and discharges include those made by or into the justice system, the police or alcohol and drug rehabilitation services.
- *Secondary health care* includes referrals and discharges made from or to (non-psychiatric) hospitals, accident and emergency services, public health services and community support services.
- *Education* referrals and discharges include those made from or to education providers, vocational services and mental health community skills enhancement programmes.
- *Others and unknown* includes referrals and discharges made from or into the social welfare system, services not already listed plus unknown sources or destinations.

Source: Programme for the Integration of Mental Health Data (PRIMHD).

StatLink http://dx.doi.org/10.1787/888933845453

Community services provide a good opportunity for better-integrated support

There are various social and community services available in New Zealand for young people experiencing mental health problems. Perhaps the foremost institutions offering support and guidance in this space are the *Youth One Stop Shops* (YOSS).

YOSS is a community-based facility offering access to health (including mental health) and other services using a holistic model of care. YOSS provide targeted services to, and are responsive to the needs of, young people aged 10 to 25 years. The aim is to provide coordinated health, education, employment and social services, at little or no cost to the client. The services are strengths-based and provided in an atmosphere of trust, safety and confidentiality. The first YOSS was set-up in 1994; currently 11 such services are funded as part of the YOSS network across New Zealand and the number is still increasing.[12] The

Ministry of Health is a primary funder of these services. Additional funding is provided through a multitude of other sources such as private donors, city councils and the Ministries of Social and Youth Development.

In 2009, an evaluation of YOSS took place on request of the Ministry of Health. It consisted of a survey among 12 YOSS managers (there were 14 YOSS in 2009), 252 clients and 101 stakeholders (e.g., the Ministry, DHBs, PHOs, and other service providers) and of meetings and focus groups with approximately 50 managers and staff, 60 clients and 60 stakeholders. The evaluation focused, among other topics, on the types of services provided, the composition of the client group, reach-out to Māori communities, the effectiveness in improving access to health care, and links between YOSS and other services (Communio, 2009[30]). General health/primary care, sexual and reproductive health and family planning were the most commonly provided services (provided by 11 out of the 12 YOSS), followed by mental health services (provided by 10 YOSS). Mental health services included assessment, counselling, treatment, advocacy and support for young people with a range of mental health conditions. Eight of the 12 YOSS specifically employed a counsellor for 0.5 to 2.0 FTEs (doctors, nurses and youth workers were most commonly employed). However, it was generally reported that demand for counselling and other mental health services was clearly exceeding capacity. The eligible population per YOSS ranged from 7 000 to 54 000, and in total all YOSSs together provided services to around 28 000 to 34 000 young people. Youth aged 15-19 years most frequently visited a YOSS (52.5%), followed by the 20-24 year-olds (30%). The majority of young people (64%) were New Zealand European followed by Māori (30%).

Effectiveness in terms of improved accessibility was assessed by the opinions of managers, clients and stakeholders. Managers mentioned various ways of addressing access barriers for youth, including youth-friendly opening hours taking into account study and work commitments; service facilities located centrally and close to public transport or areas of interest to youth; mobile services to engage with youth outside the main facility; and investment in developing cultural competency skills in staff. All three survey groups thought that YOSS were very effective in helping young people receive the health service they need and quite effective in promoting access to other (non-health) services. However, as mentioned above, lacking capacity for prompt appointments with a YOSS representative or counsellor was a major barrier to better outcomes.

Concrete evidence on improvements in health and wellbeing was unavailable due to a lack of concerted data collection; the 2009 evaluation had to rely on questions posed to the three survey groups. All managers thought that YOSS were effective in helping to improve young people's health and wellbeing, and 94% of the clients and 89% of the stakeholders agreed to this. Managers stressed the importance of developing a national minimum dataset of clinical and demographic information. A renewed evaluation would be timely now, almost ten years later, given that no national data on clinical and social outcomes has been made available since. Systematic outcome measurement including information on (mental) health, education and social outcomes (such as e.g. employment success) would make a stronger case for expanding YOSS and investing in a better integration of its services with other youth services, and understanding and addressing inequities.

YOSS services were especially valued by the survey respondents for their unique focus on youth appropriateness and the creation of a collaborative environment by linking up with other service providers, which enabled primary and secondary health and social services to be integrated successfully. Of the surveyed stakeholders, almost half were linked with a YOSS by referring clients to it and 20% received referrals from a YOSS. Only few stakeholders (9%), however, provided services through a YOSS suggesting that a true integration of services is still an exemption. This especially concerns youth primary mental health services, which – back in 2009 – were seen as an important service gap by the survey respondents. A strong integration of YOSS with the parallel structure of Youth Primary Mental Health Services could contribute to further closing this gap.

Youthline and *SPARX* are two other prominent initiatives nationally available to youth with mental health conditions. *Youthline* is a charity organisation, set up in 1970, forming a collaboration of youth development organisations. Nine Youthline centres are established across New Zealand. Their main goal is to ensure that young people know where to get help and how to access support when needed. Youthline contributes to the development of leadership and personal skills in young people, and offers remote-access support (self-help programmes and a helpline operating through telephone and email) to young people experiencing mental distress. It also offers face-to-face, non-acute mental health-related support and can refer clients to clinical and social services. Youthline's mental health advice covers general wellbeing themes (self-esteem and confidence, grief and loss, life transitions or change) alongside more acute mental health-related problems like anxiety and depression, bullying, abuse and violence, self-harm and suicide. Evaluations for single Youthline centres suggest that they are well known and received but under-resourced (Research Services, 2018[31]).

SPARX is a web-based therapeutic tool to help young people experiencing mild-to-moderate depression and facing high levels of anxiety or stress. A randomised-controlled trial has shown that SPARX results in a clinically significant reduction of depression, anxiety and hopelessness and an improvement in quality of life (Merry et al., 2012[32]). As one of the initiatives under the government's Youth Mental Health Project, funding was directed at a national rollout of SPARX. An evaluation in 2016 showed that in the financial year 2014-15, 2 577 young people had registered on SPARX (in comparison, the total number of youth clients in Youth Primary Mental Health Services was 13 500). Māori, Pasifika and Asian youth were highly under-represented among SPARX users. Of all users, 82% completed at least one of the seven modules, and the share of completers was highest among those with more severe depression symptoms (Malatest International, 2016[33]). However, only 40% completed the first of the seven modules and only 24% and 10% of those went on to completing module four and seven, respectively. Reasons for not completing all SPARX modules were technical difficulties, which have meanwhile been removed (28%), no more help being needed (25%), the idea that SPARX was not helping (19%), and not liking SPARX (16%). The low adherence rates are comparable to other online mental health tools. Of the young people surveyed about their use of SPARX, 43% indicated their use for about a month, while 35% used it for a week or less. SPARX was most commonly used two or three times a week (by 42% of the respondents), followed by less than once or twice a month (32%). The Patient Health Questionnaire which is used to measure the person's mental health status is completed before using SPARX and after completion of modules four and seven (i.e. data on these three measurement points are only available for the small group who completed all these modules). The results showed an overall trend of improvement in depressive symptoms, especially for those who had more severe symptoms at the beginning. The majority of users also reported improvements in their wellbeing and the ability to manage their own wellbeing. For a slight majority, SPARX also was as an initiator to seek additional help.

To conclude, several strong community initiatives to support youth with mental health conditions are available in New Zealand. YOSS especially has great potential to further integrate (mental) health, social, educational and employment services for young people. Together with Youthline, it functions as a first point of entry from where young people can be guided quickly to additional appropriate services. Full coverage across the country would be essential and the YOSS workforce would need to be increased to be able to balance the high demand for their services remaining unmet.

Attention to and support for early school leavers

Children and young people with moderate-to-severe mental health problems are more likely to leave school early (OECD, 2015[1]). Young people who disengage from school limit their potential for gaining adequate qualifications and weaken their job opportunities. Some may disengage from the labour market and come to rely on social assistance, further weakening their mental state and increasing the burden placed on public services.

The regular pathway through education in New Zealand

Primary and secondary education in New Zealand encompass pupils aged between 5 and 19 years, with attendance being compulsory for those aged 6 to 16 years (Ministry of Education, 2017[9]).[13] School years 1-8 make up primary level education; years 9-10 lower-secondary; and years 11-13 upper-secondary level (with a possible extension into years 14 and 15 for repeaters).[14]

In 2017, some 2 500 schools in New Zealand delivered primary and secondary education to a pupil body of around 800 300 children and adolescents. State primary and secondary schools are free and accounted for 84.9% of school pupils in 2017. State schools teach the national curriculum and cater to all ethnic groups. State *integrated* schools accounted for an additional 11.2% of pupils in 2017. They deliver the national curriculum in the same way regular state schools do but apply an alternative pedagogic approach to their teaching (for example, based on a particular religious or philosophical lens) and may, in some instances, charge modest fees. The remaining 3.8% of school pupils in 2017 attended private schools and an additional 6 008 school-aged children in New Zealand were home-schooled in 2017 (Ministry of Education, 2018[15]).

New Zealand has universal enrolment in compulsory education. Enrolment in primary education has been virtually universal since at least the 1970s and enrolment in lower-secondary education has risen from around 90% in the mid-1970s to 98% today. Educational attainment at the upper-secondary level has increased steadily. Pupils in upper-secondary school study for the National Certificate of Educational Achievement (NCEA) at one of three levels corresponding to the three years of upper-secondary education (years 11-13). The share of adolescents leaving upper-secondary school with at least NCEA level 1 rose from 80.9% in 2009 to 89.4% by 2016. Meanwhile, those leaving school with at least NCEA level 2 rose from 67.5% to 80.3% and those finishing with NCEA level 3 rose from 41.9% to 53.9% (Duncanson et al., 2017[34]).

Although secondary attainment is increasing on aggregate, there remain some pockets of pupils with particularly weak outcomes. While 53.9% of school-leavers attained NCEA level 3 in 2016, on aggregate, the proportion was lower among young men (47.7%) and markedly lower among Māori and Pasifika youth (33.8% and 43.4%, respectively) (Ministry of Education, 2018[15]). Pupils from schools in poorer areas of the country also tend to achieve worse outcomes; the share of school-leavers with NCEA level 3 was only 36.5% among decile 1 schools but as high as 80.1% among decile 10 schools (Figure 3.4).

Figure 3.4. Secondary pupils in top-decile schools in New Zealand perform significantly better than their peers in low-decile schools

Educational attainment of school leavers in New Zealand by school decile, 2016

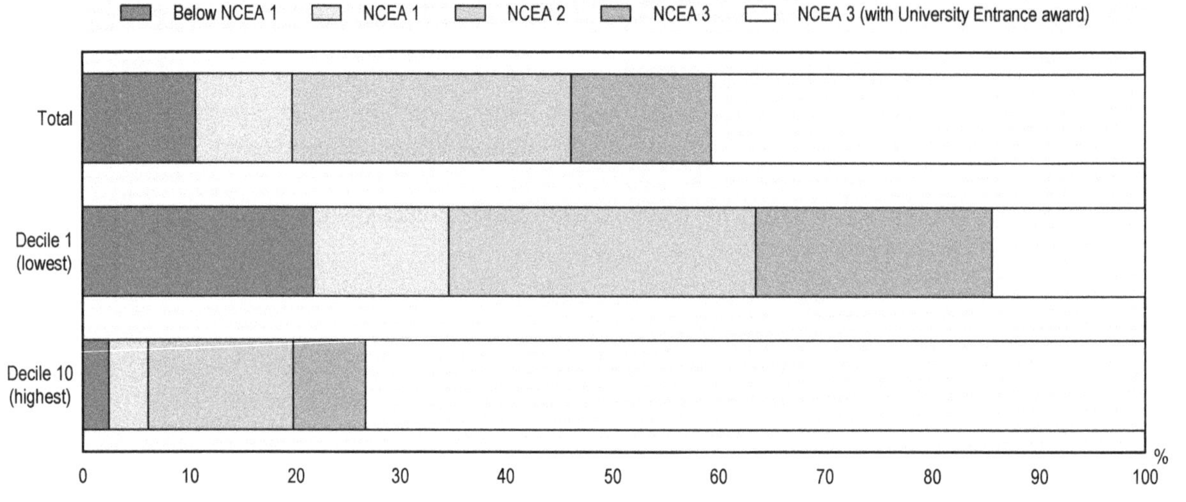

Note: NCEA=National Certificate of Educational Achievement. "School leavers" are secondary school pupils that have finished their schooling. School leavers are identified from the Ministry of Education's ENROL system, while the highest qualification status for each leaver is obtained from the New Zealand Qualifications Authority (or directly from schools for pupils attaining non-NQF qualifications).
Source: Ministry of Education (2018) *Education Works Database*.

StatLink http://dx.doi.org/10.1787/888933845472

Early school leaving programmes need a focus on mental and social issues

Early school leaving is detrimental for educational attainment and, ultimately, employment. As shown in A study from 2017 showed that NEET in New Zealand frequently use services for substance abuse and mental health conditions. Among 15-24 year-old NEETs, the share who had ever used services or treatments for substance abuse and for other mental health conditions was approximately 20% and 40%, respectively. This figure is roughly three times the proportion of youth of the same age who are still in education, and two times the level of those who are in employment. Many NEETs also received some form of social benefits during 2015: approximately 30% and 50% of males in the ages of 15-19 years and 20-24 did so, respectively, compared to about 40% and 60% of females in the same age groups . These poor social and health outcomes for NEETs demonstrate the importance of investing in the prevention of early school leaving.

Figure 3.5, almost 80% of students leaving school at age 15 end with education below NCEA 1 level, while this share drops to 40% of students leaving school at age 16. Remaining in education up until age 18 is important for achieving higher educational attainment which, in turn, increases employment opportunities, especially so for those with a mental health problem (see Chapter 1). While some early school leavers may move on to work or other training, many end up in the group of youth not in education, employment or training (NEET). In New Zealand , the share of NEET among youth aged

15-19 years and 20-24 years was 5.4% and 13.1% in 2016, respectively, just below the OECD averages of 6% and 16.2% (OECD, 2018[35]).

A study from 2017 showed that NEET in New Zealand frequently use services for substance abuse and mental health conditions. Among 15-24 year-old NEETs, the share who had ever used services or treatments for substance abuse and for other mental health conditions was approximately 20% and 40%, respectively. This figure is roughly three times the proportion of youth of the same age who are still in education, and two times the level of those who are in employment. Many NEETs also received some form of social benefits during 2015: approximately 30% and 50% of males in the ages of 15-19 years and 20-24 did so, respectively, compared to about 40% and 60% of females in the same age groups (Stats NZ, 2017[36]). These poor social and health outcomes for NEETs demonstrate the importance of investing in the prevention of early school leaving.

Figure 3.5. Educational attainment is highest for New Zealand students when they leave school at age 18

Educational attainment of school leavers in New Zealand by gender and age at which they leave, 2016

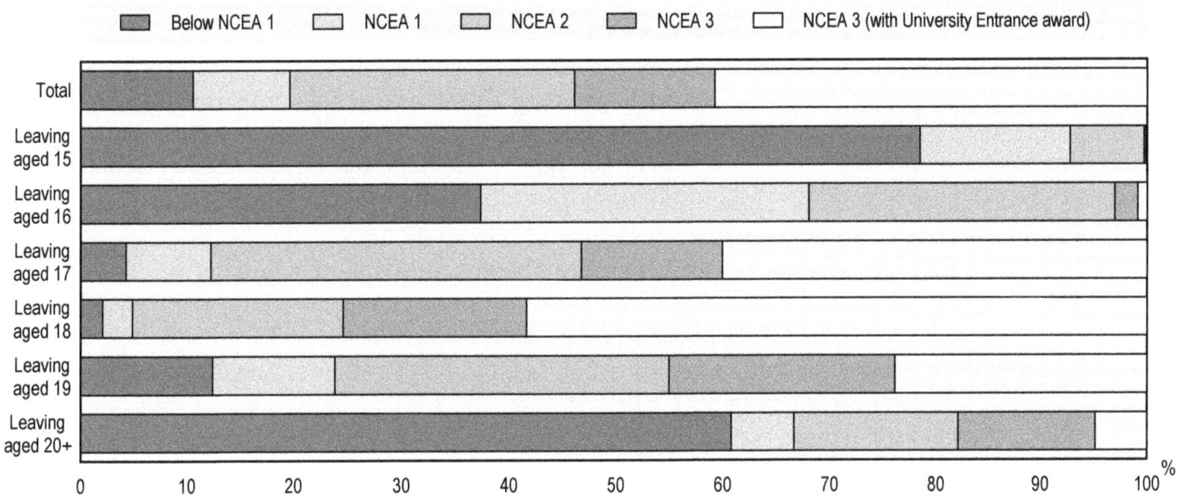

Note: NCEA=National Certificate of Educational Achievement. "School leavers" are secondary school pupils who have finished their schooling. School leavers are identified from the Ministry of Education's ENROL system, while the highest qualification status for each leaver is obtained from the New Zealand Qualifications Authority (or directly from schools for pupils attaining non-NQF qualifications).
Source: Ministry of Education (2018) *Education Works Database*.

StatLink http://dx.doi.org/10.1787/888933845491

New Zealand has a number of monitoring and support systems in place to prevent early school leaving and/or re-direct early school-leavers (or those removed from their school) back to education. Some of the most prominent institutions currently in place are: the Attendance Service; a strictly regulated Early Leaving Exemption (to prevent school suspensions and expulsions); and a variety of alternative learning pathways for vulnerable pupils including Alternative Education Programmes, Activity Centres, Teen Parent Units, Correspondence Schools and Service Academies.

The Attendance Service provides support for pupils aged 5-16 who cannot justify their absence from school. Pupils' school attendance and enrolment are monitored closely by their school, with an obligation to notify the Ministry of Education for any absence of

20 days (though the service usually engages with the pupil sooner than this) and for punitive measures like suspensions, exclusions and expulsions. The Attendance Service is delivered by a number of NGOs through an annual budget of NZD 9.6 million funded by the Ministry of Education.

In 2016, the Attendance Service received 10 854 referrals for non-attendance and 7 514 referrals for non-enrolment. Of this latter group, 47% were successfully placed into education by the end of the year; 19% were legitimately withdrawn (either because they had turned 16, moved abroad, had died or been exempted for some other valid reason); while the remaining 34% continued to received support from the Attendance Service into the following year. Non-enrolment rates vary significantly by ethnic group: while they fluctuate around two per 1 000 of the corresponding student population among European and Asian New Zealanders (age-standardised rate across all age groups), they were at eight per 1 000 in 2012 for Pasifika students (up from 4 per 1 000 in 2007) and at over 14 per 1 000 for Māori students (up from 10 per 1 000 in 2007). The link between non-enrolment and socio-economic disadvantage is strong: in 2012, students in decile 1 and 2 schools were 16 times more likely to be reported non-enrolled than students from decile 9&10 schools. Data on the link between mental health and non-enrolment are unavailable.

While school enrolment is compulsory for children and adolescents aged 6-16, the Ministry of Education may grant an Early Leaving Exemption (ELX) to pupils aged 15 who intend to pursue a promising alternative pathway.[15] An ELX may be granted only to pupils with documented problems around learning or conduct and on the condition that they would clearly benefit more from their proposed pathway than they could from school. Up to age 16, recipients of an ELX are closely monitored by the Ministry of Education – through regular contact with the employer or vocational training provider. Recipients of an ELX are eligible for *Youth Service* support under the Ministry of Social Development. There were 522 ELXs granted in 2017 (equivalent to 9.2 for every 1 000 15-year-olds in New Zealand). This is a big decrease from before 2007, when the Ministry of Education considerably strengthened its early leaving application and approval process to reduce the number of exemptions and the associated social and economic disadvantages those students were facing. Māori students have much higher rates of early leaving exemptions but the decline has affected all ethnic groups equally.

The Ministry of Education organises Alternative Education programmes (for pupils aged 13-15) and enrolment in Activity Centres (for those aged 14-17) as alternative routes through secondary education for pupils with particularly challenging behaviours or who disengage from mainstream education altogether. Alternative Education is a short-term intervention aimed at re-engaging students in a meaningful learning programme shaped to their individual needs (through an Individual Learning Plan). It supports them to transition back to school, further education, training or employment. Schools can use Activity Centres to refer students who are likely to benefit from a specialist programme meeting their social and academic needs.

In 2016, 2 872 young New Zealanders attended Alternative Education and 482 gained support from an Activity Centre – most of them boys and the biggest number identified as Māori. A review of the way at-risk pupils are supported through Alternative Education and Activity Centres concluded support is variable and generally insufficient and coming too late to make a meaningful change to young people's life choices and pathways. A main problem is adequate self-review and a lack of high-quality Individual Education

Plans. A policy tool kit available for Activity Centres to support them in adequate service delivery is rarely used (Education Review Office, 2013[37]).

Adolescents challenged with completing their schooling alongside the demands of pregnancy and early parenthood can continue their education through government-funded Teen Parent Units. Governed by mainstream high schools, these units deliver lessons based on the national curriculum alongside on-site childcare facilities, guidance and mentoring, and access to support for health, mental health and social needs. In mid-2017, Teen Parent Units supported 495 young mothers and seven young fathers throughout New Zealand. A disproportionate share of them were Māori, accounting for 61.8% of the total (Ministry of Education, 2018[15]). A recent evaluation concluded that specialised school-based services designed to meet the needs of young mothers reduce their disadvantage. Teen Parent Units are somewhat effective in raising educational enrolment and very effective in improving educational attainment (Vaithianathan et al., 2017[38]).

Children and adolescents unable to attend a local school may also engage in government-funded distance learning via the Correspondence School (now known as *Te Aho o Te Kura Pounamu*). Originally founded in 1922 to cater for around 100 children living in New Zealand's remotest parts, the Correspondence School today delivers classes to some 25 000 pupils across New Zealand (from early childhood education to secondary education) including some with specific developmental and mental health-related needs.

Learning outcomes for students in alternative forms of education stay way behind those of students in mainstream education. Of all students leaving a regular school in 2016, 56% left with NCEA 3 qualification, another 26.6% with NCEA 2 and less than 10% with below NCEA 1 (Figure 3.6). One in four students in Teen Parent Units and one in three in the Correspondence School leave school with a qualification below level 1, and only 26.7% and 16.4%, respectively, leave with NCEA 3 qualification. Outcomes for Alternative Education (for which only rough data are available) are even worse: only 37% achieve NCEA level 2 or above by age 18.

Service Academies are military-focused programmes run within secondary schools in collaboration with the New Zealand Defence Force. The Academies provide 580 places for students annually at 29 schools around New Zealand. The target group is year 12 and 13 students, particularly Māori and Pasifika males, at risk of disengaging from mainstream school who would benefit from a military-style programme. The programme offers courses in leadership and outdoor education, and is integrated with the wider school, supporting students to achieve at least NCEA level 2. An evaluation in 2011 found a high level of effectiveness of these Academies due to high quality teaching and strong leadership but also raised concerns about a lack of evidence on transitions back into regular schools and the degree to which access criteria ensure the right group of adolescents is being covered (Education Review Office, 2011[39]). The review called for stronger monitoring of the progress of students who return to school following their year in a service academy.

New Zealand has a large range of tools and options available to keep youth at risk of leaving school in education or to help those already out of school back into education. However, these programmes generally lack a focus on social and mental health issues, which may partly explain the much poorer outcomes from alternative forms of education. Social and mental health problems often play a key role among early school leavers, as shown by the situation and service use of the NEET population. Links between various 'back to education' programmes and social and mental health services are weak. Stronger interaction with available youth programmes, especially Youth One Stop Shops and

Youthline centres, which could play a bridging function, but also with Youth Primary Mental Health Services will be critical to make the system more effective. It is also crucial that resources and approaches are targeted at and led-by Māori, otherwise the inequities in outcomes will continue.

Figure 3.6. Educational attainment for New Zealand pupils varies by the type of school they have attended

Educational attainment of school leavers in New Zealand by type of school, 2016

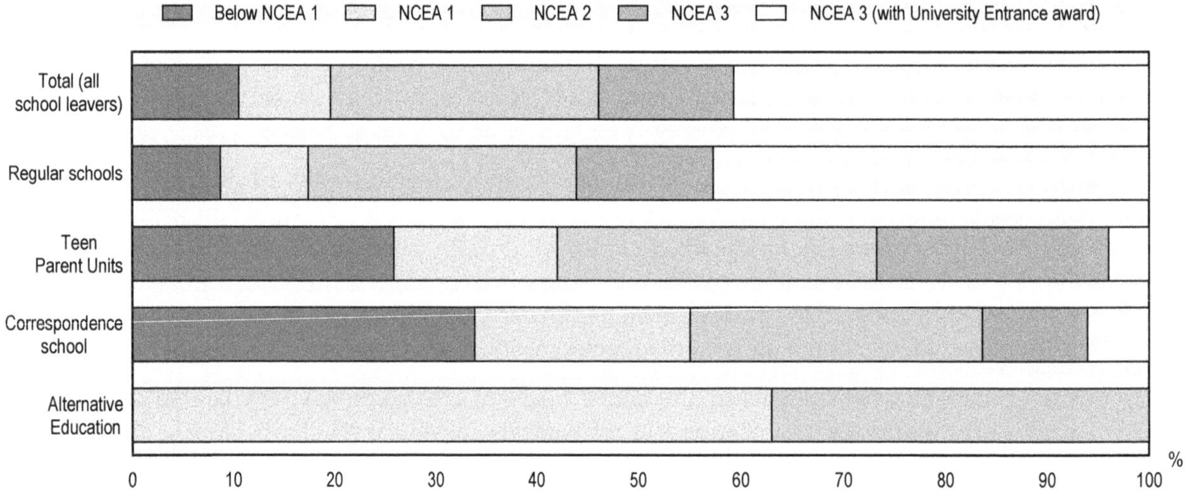

Note: NCEA=National Certificate of Educational Achievement. "School leavers" are secondary school pupils that have finished their schooling. School leavers are identified from the Ministry of Education's ENROL system, while the highest qualification status for each leaver is obtained from the New Zealand Qualifications Authority (or directly from schools for pupils attaining non-NQF qualifications).

Source: Ministry of Education (2018) *Education Works Database*.

StatLink http://dx.doi.org/10.1787/888933845510

Transitions into further education and work

The transition from secondary to tertiary education and eventually employment is challenging for many young people. In New Zealand, the youth unemployment rate is almost three times the unemployment rate of the total workforce: 12.7% versus 4.7% (OECD, 2018[40]), and the rate of Māori youth unemployment, at 21%, is even higher. Added to this, young adults with mental health problems are less likely to transition to tertiary education and face even higher joblessness compared with their peers without mental health problems (OECD, 2015[1]). Programmes and services to support young people in their transition to further education and work therefore must be able to address mental health issues adequately.

About one-third of young people in New Zealand are enrolled in some form of tertiary education, but not everyone manages to acquire a tertiary degree. For example, the great importance of completing education for good employment prospects is incontestable. Later in life, people without formal qualifications face much higher unemployment rates than their peers with tertiary qualifications (Figure 1.8, Panel A). Among those with no formal qualifications, Māori and Pasifika have much higher unemployment rates than other ethnic groups (Figure 3.8, Panel B).

The Māori and Pasifika population is also much more likely to belong to the NEET group. In 2017, the NEET rate among Māori youth aged 15-24 years was 19.5% and among Pasifika youth 17% – compared to just over 10% for European and Asian youth in New Zealand, respectively.

Figure 3.7shows that especially Māori and Pasifika students do not finish their degrees: one in three of these students drop out prematurely from their bachelor and master degree programmes, compared to one in five of students from other ethnic groups (the situation is somewhere in-between for Pasifika students in master degree programmes). Data from the National Health Survey further show that fewer young people with mental health problems reach a tertiary degree: the share of young people with a tertiary degree is 37% among those with no mental health condition compared to 33% with mild-to-moderate and 24% with severe mental health conditions, in 2016.

The great importance of completing education for good employment prospects is incontestable. Later in life, people without formal qualifications face much higher unemployment rates than their peers with tertiary qualifications (Figure 3.8, Panel A). Among those with no formal qualifications, Māori and Pasifika have much higher unemployment rates than other ethnic groups (Figure 3.8, Panel B).

The Māori and Pasifika population is also much more likely to belong to the NEET group. In 2017, the NEET rate among Māori youth aged 15-24 years was 19.5% and among Pasifika youth 17% – compared to just over 10% for European and Asian youth in New Zealand, respectively (Ministry of Business, 2017[41]).

Figure 3.7. Māori and Pasifika students drop out of higher education at much higher rates than students of other ethnic groups

Cumulative percentage of domestic full-time students who discontinued their studies by 2016 according to the year in which they have started studying, by ethnicity

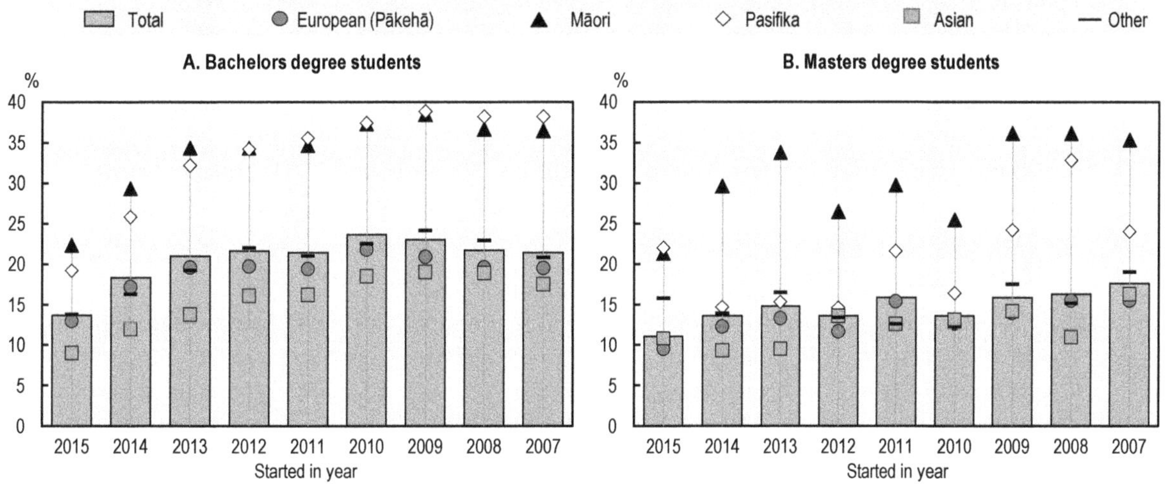

Note: Data exclude international students and part-time students.
Source: Ministry of Education (2018) *Education Works Database*.

StatLink http://dx.doi.org/10.1787/888933845529

Figure 3.8. Educational attainment and ethnicity play a key role for labour market outcomes of New Zealanders

Unemployment rate of the population aged 15 and over in New Zealand by highest qualification (Panel A) and – among the "no qualifications" group – by ethnicity (% of the labour force, Panel B)

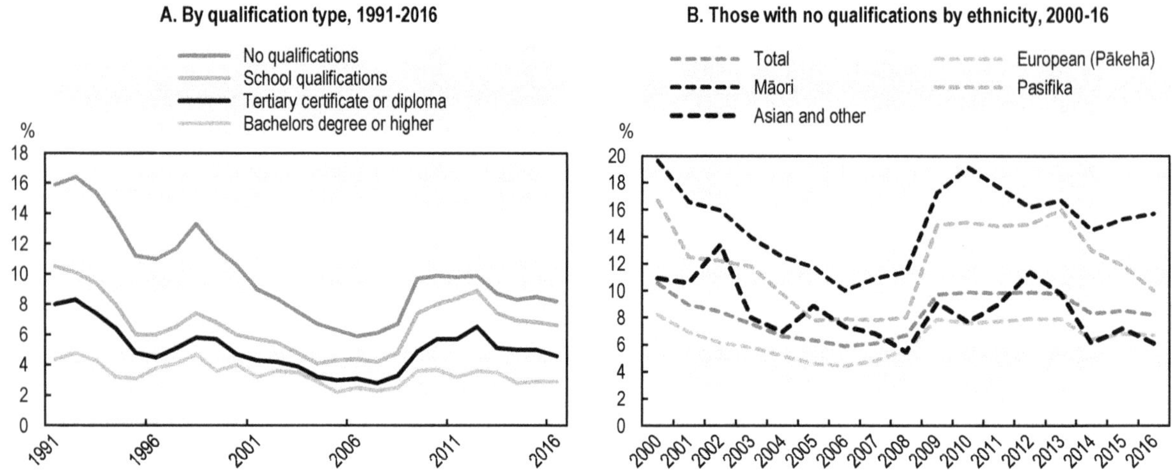

Note: "School qualifications" include NACE levels 1-3 plus equivalents from overseas. "Tertiary certificate or diplomas" include all post-secondary qualifications below bachelors-level. "No qualifications" includes an unspecified residual category in 1991-2012; 2013 estimate excludes the first quarter.
Source: Statistics New Zealand, based on *Household Labour Force Survey*.

StatLink http://dx.doi.org/10.1787/888933845548

Making the curriculum more relevant and work-oriented

New Zealand has two important structures in place to support young people in their transition to employment. One of them is the Government's Youth Guarantee. The various Youth Guarantee initiatives aim to improve the transition from school to further education and work by providing a wider range of learning opportunities, making better use of the education network and creating clear pathways from school to study and work. The New Zealand Youth Guarantee consists of six strongly interlinked initiatives: Vocational Pathways; Achievement Retention Transitions; Secondary-Tertiary Programmes; Youth Guarantee Fund (Fees Free); Secondary Tertiary Alignment Resource; and Gateway.

Vocational Pathways are structured ways for students to achieve NCEA levels 1, 2 and 3 and develop pathways to further study, training and employment. Achievement standards were developed for six key industry groups (primary industries; services industries; social and community services; manufacturing and technology; construction and infrastructure; creative industries). Students obtain a Vocational Pathways Award at NCEA level 2 when they have achieved a sufficient number of standards for one of the six industries. Vocational Pathways should increase the relevance of students' learning and provide a coherent structure for continuing education and employment. Data from 2015 showed that 29.4% of all school leavers attained NCEA level 2 with one or more Vocational Pathway Awards (O'Donnel, 2017[42]).

In 2015, the Education Review Office evaluated how well 35 secondary schools were using Vocational Pathways to provide students with a responsive and relevant curriculum. The evaluation concluded that Vocational Pathways has considerable potential to engage students in relevant learning and provide greater continuity of learning for students as they transition to further education and employment. However, at present, most schools are implementing the programme at a level that does not support this potential. Schools were aware of Vocational Pathways and included them in their careers education and course selection processes but the broader aims of increasing curriculum relevance and authenticity were less evident. In most schools, Vocational Pathways were functioning as an add-on to a traditional curriculum model, and their influence on the curriculum was thus limited. Only a few schools were using Vocational Pathways as a way of moving towards curriculum change (Holsted, 2016[43]).

Achievement Retention Transitions supports secondary schools in identifying students who may have more difficulty and, thus, need extra support in achieving NCEA level 2, and in implementing appropriate initiatives tailored to every student. The initiative specifically focuses on Māori and Pasifika students.

Secondary-Tertiary Programmes (STP) help students to remain enrolled with a secondary school while participating in various forms of education delivered by tertiary education providers. The first programmes were established in 2011, and 22 programmes have been operational since 2012. In 2014, the number of students participating in STP was 4 190, with just under 40% of participants being Māori and 14% Pasifika students. A recent evaluation of STP found mixed results. STPs have generally been effective in keeping people in education longer and increasing the number of young people who attain NCEA level 2 or equivalent and in providing pathways to employment. However, STP participants were not more likely to progress to tertiary-level education, not less likely to become NEET and there was no additional employment gain for some of the most disadvantaged groups, including especially Māori and females (Earle, 2018[44]).

Fees-free enables free-of-charge full-time study towards NCEA level 1-2 aligned with Vocational Pathways, other equivalent level 1-2 qualifications and qualifications at level 3 with tertiary education providers. It is aimed at youth aged 15-19 who have disengaged from school with no or low qualifications. The programme started in 2010 with 1 930 participants, rising to 9 000 participants by 2014. The proportion of Māori participants increased from 35% to 50% and the share of Pasifika stayed at around 20%. A recent evaluation found that Fees-free has been effective in keeping people in education and reengaging some of the NEET group. However, the programme failed to improve employment outcomes for the most disadvantaged participants, especially Māori and Pasifika participants, and being NEET and receiving a benefit was more likely for participants than for other young people with similar background (Earle, 2018[45]).

Secondary Tertiary Alignment Resource supports schools with year 11-13+ students in providing relevant learning experiences in line with Vocational Pathways to ensure a successful transition to further study and work. Schools can use extra funding to develop courses better aligned with students' needs to increase their motivation to finish education and transition smoothly to further education or work, and to provide students with opportunities to explore career pathways and take informed decisions.

Gateway enables schools to help senior students (years 11-13+) access structured workplace learning in line with Vocational Pathways (where possible). The workplace learning site needs to have a formalised learning arrangement, specified knowledge and skills for a student to attain, and specified assessment methods.

Transition support needs to be aligned with mental health and social services

The second important structure in place to support young people in their transition to employment is the Government's Youth Service. While the Youth Guarantee primarily focuses on the transition from school to higher education (and work) for youth still in education, the Youth Service, established in 2012, specifically supports the NEET group aged 16-18 years (15 year olds with an Early Leaving Exemption are also eligible), especially those receiving government payments.[16] Youth Service is a service delivered by community providers contracted by Work and Income, the operational arm of the Ministry of Social Development (MSD). The service is mandatory for those receiving government payments and voluntary for the NEET group. Youth Service providers can offer more intense and more individualised services than MSD's general employment service for adults, as they work with a caseworker-to-client ratio of one to 40. Youth Service providers are now operating in most communities.[17] Providers use the Activity Reporting Tool to monitor information and share it with MSD. Youth Service data show that from September 2012 to March 2015 the number of NEET clients rose from around 2 000 to almost 10 000. Over 75% of those clients are participating in full-time education, training or work-based training, and 50% gained NCEA credits in their first year.

Outcomes of one specific group of NEET clients, those receiving Youth Payment[18], could be compared to the group of clients who received a comparable payment before the Youth Service was in place. This comparison showed that, in the first year of benefit recipiency, 63% of the clients receiving Youth Service acquired credits and 14% reached NCEA level 2 – compared to 24% and 5%, respectively for the same clients prior to the establishment of the Youth Service (New Zealand Productivity Commission, 2015[46]). A study following Youth Service clients who receive a government payment over a period of 24-30 months also concludes that the service raises enrolment, increases education completion and, in the medium term, also improves transitions into employment (McLeod, Dixon and Crichton, 2017[47]). The impact of Youth Service support for the large and increasing group of NEETs not receiving a government payment and participating in the programme on a voluntary basis is largely unknown; presumably, good outcomes are more difficult to achieve because participants can leave the service any time without consequences or sanctions. It would be important to assess the effect of the Youth Service for this group, which is at a high risk of disengaging from education, and to explore ways to keep them in the programme.

Overall, the various interlinked initiatives under the Youth Guarantee seem to be effective in keeping young people longer in education, thereby increasing their level of educational attainment, but not very effective in raising their employment chances and lowering their NEET risk. This is especially true for the Māori population although several of the initiatives target them directly. Youth Service might deliver better employment outcomes for this group although this is difficult to establish with limited available information. As with other programmes, a key weakness of youth transition initiatives and services in New Zealand is their disconnection from other youth programmes. Better integration of the various types of supports should improve outcomes. Better integration would also imply that the right type of support can be provided earlier, which is especially critical for disadvantaged groups of the population.

Conclusion

New Zealand has an impressive array of services and institutions in place, which target schools and vulnerable students. This includes:

- the Youth One Stop Shops, a great example of an easily accessible service that combines low-threshold, integrated support with referral to specialist services;
- an effective Attendance Service to tackle and prevent early school leaving;
- various resources in schools such as additional learning supports, managing behaviour programmes and school-based health services;
- various options to complete education in an alternative way; and
- initiatives that promote the transition into work (the Youth Guarantee as well as Work and Income's Youth Service).

Many of these programmes and services are internationally of a very high standard. Actual outcomes, however, are not as impressive as the rich suite of services would seem to imply. Despite a great awareness of the need to help vulnerable students, considerable problems remain. First, Māori youth, the most disadvantaged of all groups, still have relatively poor education and employment outcomes and are over-represented among all groups at risk – such as early school leavers and NEETs – and among users of most services, while also being the group with the highest mental health prevalence. Most initiatives and supports show poorer effectiveness for Māori youth, including some especially targeted for them. This this warrants a better understanding of the reasons why the targeted approach was ineffective, in order to ensure (more) equal outcomes for all groups in the future.

Secondly, many services and initiatives are insufficiently resourced and many have to draw their resources from several government and non-government donors. Most initiatives are initially set-up as an experiment and many remain in a trial phase for years if not forever. Trials rarely cover the entire country and even if a service is rolled-out nationally, it appears that the accessibility and availability of supports varies considerably across the country. More national guidance and monitoring would be an important step to ensure all youth across New Zealand can benefit from the best available service.

Thirdly, it appears that the links and transitions between many of the services and institutions are underdeveloped. This has multiple consequences, including duplication of service, lacking referrals to the appropriate service and unnecessary delays in getting the right service. For the user, i.e. for the youth population, it will not always be clear where (best) to go and the outcome may be highly path-dependant. Improving this situation will require more of a nation-wide public policy and clearer political leadership.

Finally, most initiatives and services lack sufficient attention to mental health, including all non-medical youth services but also most school-based health services and even the before-school health check. This has significant consequences later on because children's' and adolescents' mental health problems are often the cause of poor outcomes later and underlying the substantial inequities.

The government is currently developing a wider, cross-government and cross-agency NEET strategy. The strategy aims to: i) raise the proportion of school-age people who remain in education and complete their NCEA level 2 qualification; ii) reduce the flow from the schooling system to NEET status; iii) invest in activating the existing stock of young people in the NEET group; and iv) reduce the number of young people dependent on government payments. For this strategy to succeed it will be crucially important to recognise why support hitherto provided has not improved youth outcomes sufficiently and to address the programme and system weaknesses identified in this report.

Notes

[1] Recognition of the key competencies emerged from the recommendations produced under the OECD's Definition and Selection of Competencies (*DeSeCo*) project (OECD, 2005[56])

[2] While the key competencies mainstream mental wellbeing throughout pupils' school experience, the stand-alone subject of Health and Physical Education (HPE) provides explicit teaching on mental health to pupils in secondary schools (http://health.tki.org.nz/). The Health component of HPE covers mental health as a learning programme alongside sexuality, food and nutrition, body care and physical safety. Most secondary schools teach HPE on a compulsory basis to lower-secondary school pupils in years 9 and 10. Upper-secondary school pupils in years 11-13 can choose to continue studying HPE as one of their elective subjects. In 2016, 15% of upper-secondary school pupils were studying either HPE or the health component of HPE on its own (Ministry of Education, 2018[15]).

[3] The ERO is a public body tasked with evaluating and reporting on the education and care of pupils in school (and pre-school). In recent years, ERO has increased its attention on the key competencies and, more generally, pupils' wellbeing (Education Review Office, 2016[58]).

[4] Schools can issue stand-downs, suspensions, exclusions or expulsions. Pupils issued with a stand-down are formally sent home from school for up to five school days. Those issued with a suspension are also formally sent home from school but require a decision from the school's management board to return or expel them (in 2016, schools decided in 62% of cases to lift a suspension rather than expel the pupil). A pupil issued with an exclusion or an expulsion is dis-enrolled from the school and supported to enrol elsewhere within a period of 10 days.

[5] Male pupils are three times more likely than female students to receive a stand-down, suspension or exclusion and over four times more likely to be expelled. Differences by ethnic groups are of a similar magnitude. For instance, in 2016 Māori pupils were issued 2.4 times as many stand-downs as European (*Pākehā*) pupils, 3.3 times as many suspensions and 3.4 times as many exclusions, and 3.6 times many expulsions (Ministry of Education, 2018[15]). Pasifika youth are found between the two groups except for expulsions, which affected them more often than any other group.

[6] Under the PB4L initiative, New Zealand also operates a comprehensive programme with integrated services to empower young people to enjoy a successful life, the *Intensive Wraparound Service*. It targets children with complex mental health, behavioural and special learning needs, a challenge outside the scope of this report; but the holistic wraparound approach offers a number of lessons and has shown equally strong outcomes for Māori children (Burgon, Berg and Herdina, 2015[59])

[7] New Zealand's schools are currently sorted into funding deciles according to a composite index of five socio-economic variables, updated every five years via the population and housing census. Categorisation relates to the geographic areas from which schools obtain their pupils. Funding deciles are determined according to: a) the share of households in the lowest income quintile (adjusted for age); b) the share of employed parents in low-skill occupations; c) the share of households with high crowding (according to a ratio between occupants and bedrooms, adjusted for age and coupledom); d) the share of parents by educational attainment; and e) the share of parents who directly claimed income support during the previous year.

[8] In some areas, Public Health Units or DHBs also provide health nursing in schools, including primary and intermediate schools. Their services vary according to school need and generally range from visits once a week to once a school term. Some secondary schools have both services in place.

[9] Initiatives led by the Ministry of Health include: 1) expansion of school-based health services to more low-decile schools; 2) roll-out of the HEADS Assessment in schools and primary care settings; 3) expansion of primary mental health services for age group 12-19; 4) introduction of an online therapy tool called *SPARX*; 5) better responsiveness of primary care to young people's mental health (including funding for Youth One Stop Shops); 6-7) improvements in follow-up care and access under the child and adolescent mental health services and youth alcohol and drug services. Initiatives led by the Ministry of Education include: 8-10) programmes under the broader PB4L initiative; 11) ERO's *Wellbeing for Success* review and support tools; 12) an ERO review of the school guidance system; 13) a review of Alcohol and Other Drug Education Services. Initiatives led by the Ministry of Social Development include: 14) placing social workers in low-decile secondary schools; 15) a new social media innovation fund (known as *Lifehack*); 16) improvements in the "youth-friendliness" of common online mental health resources; 17) better access to information for parents, families and friends (including the *Common Ground* initiative); 18) temporary funding for Youth One Stop Shops (now concluded); 19) a review of referral pathways into youth mental health services; 20) initiatives to engage young people in the Youth Mental Health Project; 21) initiatives to improve school attendance among young people with mental health issues. Initiatives led by Te Puni Kōkiri include: 22) *Whānau Ora* ("family health") for Youth Mental Health; 23) support for new referral pathways into youth mental health services; 24) development of integrated funding models and better connected services; 25) co-location of additional social services in schools. Finally, there is one regional initiative 26) for youth mental health in Canterbury.

[10] Total spending for the Social Workers in Schools services is around NZD 21.4 million per year, corresponding to about NZD 35 000 for every school supported by the programme.

[11] Since March 2018, a new school-based initiative in several school clusters across Canterbury (Mana Ake – Stronger for Tomorrow) offers early intervention and support for teachers, families and whanau when children are experiencing ongoing issues that affect their wellbeing. The Mana Ake provider network offers a range of skills, including psychologists, social workers, counsellors and youth workers (see http://ccn.health.nz/FocusAreas/ManaAke-StrongerforTomorrow.aspx).

[12] Youth One-Stop Shops include the *Anamata Café for Youth Health* in Taupo; the *Directions Youth Health Centre* for Hastings and Napier; *Evolve* in Wellington; *Kapiti Youth Support* in Kapiti Coast; the *Korowai Youth Well-being Trust* in Christchurch; *Number 10* in Invercargill; *Rotovegas* in Rotorua; *Vibe* for Lower Hutt and Upper Hutt; the *Whangarei Youth Space* in Whangarei; the *Youth One Stop Shop* in Palmerston North; and the *Youth Services Trust* in Whanganui.

[13] Note that secondary school in New Zealand was only mandatory up to the age of 15 until 1989. Since then, it has been age 16.

[14] Note that virtually all infants in New Zealand take part in early childhood education (i.e. pre-primary education). Some 4 000 certified operators provide early childhood education including education and care centres, kindergartens, play centres and Māori-language centres called *kōhanga reo* (Ministry of Education, 2017$_{[9]}$). Enrolment at the pre-primary level is higher than in most other OECD countries, with early childhood education encompassing 65% of 2-year-olds, 89% of three-year-olds and 94% of four-year-olds – compared with respective OECD averages of 54%, 78% and 87% (OECD, 2017$_{[60]}$). Although pre-primary education is outside the scope of this report, it is an equally important place to support the mental development and resilience of children, and identify and address early signs of mental health problems.

[15] See: www.education.govt.nz/school/student-support/early-leaving-exemption/.

[16] In June 2017, there were 171 409 New Zealanders 0-17 year olds dependent on a benefit. Most of these children and young people (118 384 or 69%) were reliant on a recipient of sole parent support, with the remainder was reliant on recipients of jobseeker support (32 055 or 19%), supported living payments (18 027 or 11%) or other benefits (2 943 or 2%).

[17] In most parts of the country, MSD contracts only one Youth Service provider in each community (only in Wellington and Whanganui, in-house MSD caseworkers provide the service themselves). Providers hold outcome-based contracts to improve the proportions of young people in education, training and employment. They receive an administration fee upfront; a further third of possible payments for achievement of milestones, such as enrolling in education; and a bonus third for the client completing specified results, such as gaining a NCEA certificate. Youth Service replaces the former Youth Transition Service operated in some MSD offices but without uniform design.

[18] The Youth Payment is a financial support measure for young people aged 16 or 17 who cannot live with their parents or guardian and do not receive any supported from them or anyone else.

References

(n.a.)((n.d.)), *School Evaluation Indicators: Effective Practice for Improvement and Learner Success.* [57]

Bernay, R. et al. (2016), "Pause, breathe, smile: a mixed-methods study of student well-being following participation in an eight-week, locally developed mindfulness program in three New Zealand schools", *Advances in School Mental Health Promotion*, Vol. 9/2, pp. 90-106, http://dx.doi.org/10.1080/1754730X.2016.1154474. [17]

Best Practice Advocacy Centre New Zealand (2015), "Addressing mental health and wellbeing in young people", *Best Practice Journal*, Vol. 71, https://bpac.org.nz/BPJ/2015/October/docs/BPJ71-wellbeing.pdf (accessed on 07 February 2018). [20]

Boyd, S., L. Bonne and M. Berg (2017), *Finding a balance—fostering student wellbeing, positive behaviour, and learning: Findings from the NZCER national survey of primary and intermediate schools 2016*, New Zealand Council for Educational Research, Wellington, http://www.nzcer.org.nz/system/files/National%20Survey_Wellbeing_for%20publication_0.pdf (accessed on 20 February 2018). [12]

Burgon, J., M. Berg and N. Herdina (2015), *Patterns of student progress in the Intensive Wraparound Service: NZCER IWS Evaluation Report*, Ministry of Education, Wellington, http://www.educationcounts.govt.nz/publications.. [59]

Clark, T. et al. (2013), *Youth'12 Overview: The Health and Wellbeing of New Zealand Secondary School Students in 2012*, University of Auckland, Auckland, https://www.fmhs.auckland.ac.nz/assets/fmhs/faculty/ahrg/docs/2012-overview.pdf (accessed on 31 January 2018). [2]

Communio (2009), *Evaluation of Youth One Stop Shops: Final report*, Ministry of Health, https://www.health.govt.nz/system/files/documents/publications/youth-one-stop-shop-evaluation-report-v1.1.pdf. [30]

Cooper, K. and K. Stewart (2015), *Does Money in Adulthood Affect Adult Outcomes?*, Joseph Rowntree Foundation, York, http://www.jrf.org.uk/sites/default/files/jrf/migrated/files/money-adult-outcomes-full.pdf (accessed on 27 October 2018). [6]

Denny S., T. et al. (2014), *Health Services in New Zealand Secondary Schools and the Associated Health Outcomes for Students The Health and Wellbeing of New Zealand Secondary School Students in 2012 Title: Health Services in New Zealand Secondary Schools and the Associated Health Outcomes for Students*, University of Auckland, Auckland, https://cdn.auckland.ac.nz/assets/fmhs/faculty/ahrg/docs/Youth%20%E2%80%9912%20Health%20Services%20and%20Health%20Outcomes.pdf (accessed on 27 June 2018). [22]

Devcich, D. et al. (2017), "Effectiveness of a Mindfulness-Based Program on School Children's Self-Reported Well-Being: A Pilot Study Comparing Effects With An Emotional Literacy Program", *Journal of Applied School Psychology*, Vol. 33/4, pp. 309-330, http://dx.doi.org/10.1080/15377903.2017.1316333. [18]

Duncanson, M. et al. (2017), *Child poverty monitor: 2017 Technical Report*, New Zealand Child and Youth Epidemiology Service, University of Otago, http://dx.doi.org/10.1007/s12187-015-9357-8. [34]

Durie, M. (2002), "Universal provision, indigeneity and the Treaty of Waitangi", *Victoria University Wellington Law Review*, Vol. 33, https://heinonline.org/hol-cgi-bin/get_pdf.cgi?handle=hein.journals/vuwlr33&section=31 (accessed on 12 October 2018). [54]

Earle, D. (2018), *Secondary-Tertiary Programmes: Monitoring Youth Guarantee 2017*, Ministry of Education, Wellington, https://www.educationcounts.govt.nz/__data/assets/pdf_file/0009/184752/Monitoring-Youth-Guarantee-2017-Secondary-Tertiary-Programmes.pdf (accessed on 30 June 2018). [44]

Earle, D. (2018), *Youth Guarantee Fees-Free places: Monitoring Youth Guarantee 2017*, Ministry of Education, Wellington, https://www.educationcounts.govt.nz/__data/assets/pdf_file/0008/184751/Monitoring-Youth-Guarantee-2017-Youth-Guarantee-Fees-Free-places.pdf (accessed on 30 June 2018). [45]

Education Review Office (2016), *Effective Internal Evaluation for Improvement*, Education Review Office, Wellington, http://www.ero.govt.nz/assets/Uploads/Effective-internal-evaluation-for-improvement.pdf (accessed on 05 February 2018). [14]

Education Review Office (2016), *School Evaluation Indicators: Effective Practice for Improvement and Learner Success*, Education Review Office, Wellington, http://www.ero.govt.nz/assets/Uploads/ERO-15968-School-Evaluation-Indicators-2016-v10lowres.pdf. [58]

Education Review Office (2015), *Wellbeing for Children's Success at Primary School*, Education Review Office, Wellington, http://www.ero.govt.nz/assets/Uploads/ERO-Wellbeing-Primary-Schools-WEB.pdf (accessed on 20 February 2018). [13]

Education Review Office (2013), *Provision for Students in Activity Centres*, Education Review Office, Wellington, http://www.ero.govt.nz/assets/Uploads/Provision-for-Students-in-Activity-Centres-June-2013-cover.pdf (accessed on 30 June 2018). [37]

Education Review Office (2013), *Wellbeing for Success: Draft Evaluation Indicators for Student Wellbeing*, Education Review Office, Wellington, http://www.ero.govt.nz/assets/Uploads/Wellbeing-For-Success.pdf (accessed on 01 February 2018). [8]

Education Review Office (2011), *An Evaluation of Service Academies*, Education Review Office, Wellington, http://www.ero.govt.nz/assets/Uploads/An-Evaluation-of-Services-Academies-September-2011.pdf (accessed on 30 June 2018). [39]

Gibson, K. et al. (2017), *Child poverty and mental health A literature review*, The New Zealand Psychological Society Inc., Auckland, http://www.cpag.org.nz (accessed on 27 October 2018). [5]

Gluckman, P. (2011), *Improving the Transition: Reducing Social and Psychological Morbidity During Adolescence - A report from the Prime Minister's Chief Science Advisor*, Office of the Prime Minister's Science Advisory Committee, Wellington, http://www.pmcsa.org.nz (accessed on 28 February 2018). [21]

Gustavsson, A. et al. (2011), "Cost of disorders of the brain in Europe 2010.", *European neuropsychopharmacology : the journal of the European College of Neuropsychopharmacology*, Vol. 21/10, pp. 718-79, http://dx.doi.org/10.1016/j.euroneuro.2011.08.008. [48]

Hipkins, R. (2006), *The Nature of the Key Competencies: A Background Paper*, New Zealand Council for Educational Research, Wellington, http://www.nzcer.org.nz/system/files/nature-of-k-round-paper.pdf (accessed on 05 February 2018). [10]

Ho, F. et al. (2016), "The Efficacy and Cost-Effectiveness of Stepped Care Prevention and Treatment for Depressive and/or Anxiety Disorders: A Systematic Review and Meta-Analysis.", *Scientific reports*, Vol. 6, p. 29281, http://dx.doi.org/10.1038/srep29281. [26]

Holsted, I. (2016), *Vocational Pathways: Authentic and Relevant Learning*, Education Review Office, Wellington, http://www.ero.govt.nz/assets/Uploads/Vocational-Pathways-PDF2.pdf (accessed on 30 June 2018). [43]

Macdonald, J. et al. (2015), *My FRIENDS Youth: final evaluation report Report to the Ministry of Education*, Ministry of Education, Wellington, http://www.nzcer.org.nz/system/files/My-FRIENDS-Youth-final-evaluation-report.pdf (accessed on 28 June 2018). [24]

Malatest International (2016), *Evaluation of SPARX*, https://www.health.govt.nz/system/files/documents/publications/evaluation-sparx-dec16.pdf. [33]

Malatest International (2016), *Evaluation Report: The Youth Primary Mental Health Service*, Ministry of Health, https://www.health.govt.nz/system/files/documents/publications/evaluation-report-youth-primary-mental-health-service-dec16.pdf. [27]

Mane, J. (2009), "Kaupapa Māori: A community approach", *MAI Review*, Vol. 3/1, http://review.mai.ac.nz (accessed on 12 October 2018). [53]

McLeod, K., S. Dixon and S. Crichton (2017), "Evaluation of the impact of the Youth Service: Youth Payment and Young Parent Payment", The Treasury, Wellington, https://treasury.govt.nz/publications/wp/evaluation-impact-youth-service-youth-payment-and-young-parent-payment-wp-16-07-html (accessed on 27 October 2018). [47]

Medibank and Nous Group (2013), *The Case for Mental Health Reform in Australia: A Review of Expenditure and System Design*, Medibank Private Limited and Nous Group, https://www.medibank.com.au/client/documents/pdfs/the_case_for_mental_health_reform_in_australia.pdf (accessed on 05 June 2018). [49]

Mental Health Commission (1998), *Blueprint for mental health services in New Zealand: How things need to be*, Mental Health Commission, Wellington, http://www.worldcat.org/title/blueprint-for-mental-health-services-in-new-zealand-how-things-need-to-be/oclc/154672995 (accessed on 01 March 2018). [29]

Merry, S. et al. (2012), "The effectiveness of SPARX, a computerised self help intervention for adolescents seeking help for depression: randomised controlled non-inferiority trial.", *BMJ (Clinical research ed.)*, Vol. 344, p. e2598, http://dx.doi.org/10.1136/BMJ.E2598. [32]

Ministry of Business, I. (2017), *Not in employment, education and training*, http://www.mbie.govt.nz/info-services/employment-skills/labour-market-reports/pacific-peoples-labour-market-trends/march-2017/neet (accessed on 30 June 2018). [41]

Ministry of Education (2018), *Education Counts Database*, Statistics, https://www.educationcounts.govt.nz/statistics (accessed on 07 February 2018). [15]

Ministry of Education (2017), *New Zealand Education System: Overview*, New Zealand Government, Wellington, https://www.education.govt.nz/assets/Uploads/NZ-Education-System-Overview-publication-web-format.pdf (accessed on 29 January 2018). [9]

Ministry of Education (2007), *The New Zealand Curriculum*, New Zealand Government, Wellington, http://nzcurriculum.tki.org.nz/The-New-Zealand-Curriculum (accessed on 01 February 2018). [11]

Ministry of Health (2016), *Suicide Facts: Deaths and intentional self-harm.* [4]

Ministry of Social Development (2015), *Guidelines: Supporting young people with stress, anxiety and/or depression*, Ministry of Social Development, Wellington, http://www.msd.govt.nz/documents/about-msd-and-our-work/publications-resources/brochures/supporting-young-people-stress-anxiety-depression.pdf (accessed on 07 February 2018). [19]

New Zealand Productivity Commission (2015), *More effective social services*, ew Zealand Productivity Commission, Wellington, https://www.productivity.govt.nz/sites/default/files/social-services-final-report-main.pdf (accessed on 30 June 2018). [46]

O'Donnel, S. (2017), *Upper Secondary Education in New Zealand: Full Review*, https://www.ncca.ie/media/3333/new-zealand-full-review-3.pdf (accessed on 30 June 2018). [42]

OECD (2018), *Youth not in employment, education or training (NEET)*, Youth and the labour market, https://doi.org/10.1787/7b765a3b-en. [35]

OECD (2018), *Youth unemployment rate (indicator)*, https://doi.org/10.1787/c3634df7-en (accessed on 30 June 2018). [40]

OECD (2017), *Back to Work: New Zealand: Improving the Re-employment Prospects of Displaced Workers*, Back to Work, OECD Publishing, Paris, http://dx.doi.org/10.1787/9789264264434-en. [51]

OECD (2017), *Education at a glance: OECD indicators*, http://www.oecd-ilibrary.org/education/education-at-a-glance-2017_eag-2017-en. [60]

OECD (2017), *Indicator CO4.4 Teenage suicides (15-19 years old)*, OECD Family Database, https://www.oecd.org/els/family/CO_4_4_Teenage-Suicide.pdf (accessed on 03 July 2018). [3]

OECD (2017), *PISA 2015 Results (Voluime III): Student's Well-Being*, PISA, OECD Publishing, https://www.oecd.org/pisa/PISA-2015-Results-Students-Well-being-Volume-III-Overview.pdf (accessed on 27 June 2018). [16]

OECD (2015), *Fit Mind, Fit Job: From Evidence to Practice in Mental Health and Work*, Mental Health and Work, OECD Publishing, Paris, http://dx.doi.org/10.1787/9789264228283-en. [1]

OECD (2015), *Fit Mind, Fit Job: From Evidence to Practice in Mental Health and Work*, Mental Health and Work, OECD Publishing, Paris, http://dx.doi.org/10.1787/9789264228283-en. [52]

OECD (2015), *Recommendation of the Council on Integrated Mental Health, Skills and Work Policy*, OECD Publications, Paris, https://legalinstruments.oecd.org/Instruments/ShowInstrumentView.aspx?InstrumentID=334&Lang=en&Book=False (accessed on 08 February 2018). [7]

OECD (2012), *Sick on the Job?: Myths and Realities about Mental Health and Work*, Mental Health and Work, OECD Publishing, Paris, http://dx.doi.org/10.1787/9789264124523-en. [55]

OECD (2005), *The Definition and Selection of Key competencies: Executive Summary*, OECD Publishing, Paris, https://www.oecd.org/pisa/35070367.pdf. [56]

Office of the Health and Disability Commissioner (2018), *New Zealand's mental health and addiction services: The monitoring and advocacy report of the Mental Health Commissioner*, Office of the Health and Disability Commissioner, Wellington, http://www.hdc.org.nz/media/4688/mental-health-commissioners-monitoring-and-advocacy-report-2018.pdf (accessed on 02 March 2018). [28]

RANZCP (2016), *The economic cost of serious mental illness and comorbidities in Australia and New Zealand*, Royal Australian and New Zealand College of Psychiatrists, Melbourne, https://www.ranzcp.org/Files/Publications/RANZCP-Serious-Mental-Illness.aspx (accessed on 05 June 2018). [50]

Research Services (2018), *Evaluation of Youthline Wellington: Qualitative Exploration*, Youthline Wellington, Wellington, http://www.communityresearch.org.nz/wp-content/uploads/formidable/8/REPORT-EVALUATION-OF-YOUTHLINE-WELLINGTON.pdf (accessed on 28 June 2018). [31]

Stats NZ (2017), *Otago youth not in employment, education, or training (NEET): Collaborative research between Stats NZ and Methodist Mission Southern using integrated data.*, Retrieved from www.stats.govt.nz, Wellington, https://www.stats.govt.nz/assets/Reports/Otago-youth-not-in-employment-education-or-training-NEET/otago-youth-neet-2015-report.pdf (accessed on 28 June 2018). [36]

Superu (2016), *The Prime Minister's Youth Mental Health Project: SUMMATIVE EVALUATION REPORT*, Social Policy Evaluation Unit, Wellington, http://www.superu.govt.nz/sites/default/files/YMHP%20Summative%20Report%202016.pdf (accessed on 28 June 2018). [23]

Vaithianathan, R. et al. (2017), "IMPACT OF SCHOOL-BASED SUPPORT ON EDUCATIONAL OUTCOMES OF TEEN-MOTHERS: EVIDENCE FROM NEW ZEALAND'S TEEN PARENT UNITS", Ministry of Social Development, Wellington, https://www.msd.govt.nz/documents/about-msd-and-our-work/publications-resources/working-papers/wp-02-24-teen-parent-unit-impact-study-working-paper.pdf (accessed on 27 October 2018). [38]

Wilson, M. et al. (2018), "Estimating the impact of Social Workers in Schools using linked administrative data", Ministry of Social Development and Ministry for Children, Wellington, http://www.stats.govt.nz. (accessed on 27 October 2018). [25]

Chapter 4. Addressing mental health in New Zealand's workplaces

This chapter reviews policies, programmes and activities of key stakeholders involved in promoting mental wellbeing within New Zealand's workplaces and retaining workers who experience mental health problems. The analysis looks, in particular, at the common ways in which employers manage mental health risks and address concerns when they emerge; how public campaigns combat stigma, discrimination and misconceptions surrounding mental health; how New Zealand helps workers with mental health problems reintegrate into the labour market; and how sickness leave policies help or hinder them. Throughout this chapter, the analysis draws upon the OECD Council Recommendation on Integrated Mental Health, Skills and Work Policy *of 2015 as the primary benchmark for best practices in this field.*

Introduction

The links between mental health and work are multi-fold. With one in five workers at any moment experiencing mental health conditions in all OECD countries, workplaces have to deal with these problems and their consequences on a daily basis. In view of this, the pervasiveness of mental health stigma in the workplace is surprising. Many employers would not hire even highly qualified applicants if they knew they had a mental health condition. Not surprisingly, therefore, many employees with mental illness choose not to disclose because they fear discrimination and dismissal.

This confused situation is problematic for several reasons. First, unrecognised or unsupported mental health conditions are very costly for employers through longer sickness absences of these workers and higher productivity losses while at work. Secondly, longer and repeated periods of sick leave are often a steppingstone to labour market exit and permanent inactivity. This is especially problematic in view of the increasing evidence that employment is generally good for mental health, and can speed up recovery. But this is not necessarily true in every situation because poor-quality jobs, poor leadership, and psychosocial stress in the workplace can put mental health under strain and exacerbate underlying mental health problems (OECD, 2015[1]).

New Zealand has only limited data to measure these manifold associations and implications. A 2016 survey by Business New Zealand based on a relatively small sample of companies finds that businesses lost an estimated 6.6 million working days in 2016 due to sickness absence (an average of 4.4 days per worker), costing the economy around NZD 1.5 billion per year (BusinessNZ and Southern Cross Health Society, 2017[2]). The extent to which this loss is due to mental illness is unknown but the survey findings indicate rising levels of work-related stress and a high degree of presenteeism among workers (i.e. people underperforming at work because of health issues). Another survey of working-age adults, also in 2016, points to a reluctance to disclose mental distress, especially in work settings (Health Promotion Agency, 2018[3]).

These findings and the underlying dynamics call for strong efforts by employers to identify and prevent psychosocial risks at work and respond to mental health problems of their workers. These efforts need matching by the New Zealand government to support employers in their tasks and provide regulations, guidance and tools to help workers with mental illness keep their jobs. This chapter analyses how these issues are approached in New Zealand, what could be improved and what the country could learn from promising approaches in other OECD countries.

The main challenges for New Zealand's workplace policies

The OECD *Recommendation of the Council on Integrated Mental Health, Skills and Work Policy* calls upon its member countries to: "seek to develop and implement policies for workplace mental health promotion and return-to-work in close dialogue and co-operation with the social partners," detailing several key priorities for action that policy makers should consider (OECD, 2015[4]).

Table 4.1 gives a brief assessment of New Zealand's performance in each of these policy areas, and suggested actions. In summary, the situation is as follows:

Table 4.1. New Zealand's performance regarding the OECD Council Recommendations around improving workplace mental health promotion and return-to-work

	OECD Council Recommendation	New Zealand's performance	Suggested actions
A	Promote and enforce **psychosocial risk assessment and risk prevention in the workplace** consistent with applicable privacy and non-discrimination laws, to ensure that all companies comply with their responsibilities.	Information on workplace stress and bullying is still limited and knowledge on what to do is underdeveloped Health and safety legislation is still seen as safety oriented; enforcement in terms of work-related health is poor WorkSafe (the lead health and safety regulator) lacks financial resources and sufficient psychosocial risk competence to support businesses in managing health and safety risks	Enforce legislation through obligations for employers (e.g. prevention plans) and corresponding support (e.g. guidance tools that describe risks) and sanction those who do not comply Train WorkSafe staff on psychosocial issues, strengthen its enforcement capacity (e.g. implement workplace measures) and increase its resources Review the effectiveness of legislation and WorkSafe capacity building
B	Develop a strategy for **addressing stigma, discrimination and misconceptions** faced by workers living with mental health conditions at their workplace, with a focus on leadership and improved competencies of managers and worker representatives to deal with mental health issues.	Toolkits for employers, such as Open Minds, developed by various mental health agencies Employer Advice Line (Monday to Friday telephone service) High workplace bullying prevalence due in part to high job insecurity and depressed wages Significant employer-led initiatives and networks	Evaluate the reach and impact of toolkits, also in small and medium-sized enterprises and disseminate available toolkits widely Improve focus on quality work and stress prevention in collective agreements Share good practices of employers and employer networks, involving especially smaller enterprises
C	Promote greater **awareness of the potential labour productivity losses due to mental health conditions** by developing guidelines for line managers, human resource professionals and worker representatives to stimulate a better response to workers' mental health conditions.	Relatively short period of sick pay, also implying high presenteeism Employers often lack the skills and knowledge to address mental health problems of their workers Employee Assistance Programmes (EAP) available in larger companies, but covering less than one in three workers across the country System of occupational health is underdeveloped/focused on safety	Invest in good evidence base and collect key data in a systematic way Increase period of employer-paid sick leave to stimulate healthy workplaces Ensure EAPs are widely available in small and medium-sized companies, regulate minimum standards and facilitate EAP contracts Single point of contact for employers to receive support and guidance in dealing with mental health matters Help companies access and implement good practices
D	Foster the design of structured **return-to-work policies and processes** for workers on sick leave and their employers, and encourage a dialogue between the sick worker, the employer and the involved health practitioners.	Limited focus on return to work after sickness, and no public return-to-work support or strategy A unique Accident Compensation system (ACC) with a range of undesirable side effects especially for stress-related illnesses and mental health conditions – a no-fault system with a strict illness-injury boundary	Promote return-to-work strategies with mutual obligations for all actors Replicate the comprehensive ACC approach and process for cases of illness ("learn from ACC") Consider expanding ACC to cover illness, as intended in the past

Source: Authors' own assessment based on all of the evidence collected in this chapter.

New Zealand is making great headway in developing cutting-edge, integrated national datasets but there are gaps in information on workplace health outcomes. Data on sickness absence are not nationally routinely collected in any way. This must change as good policy-making relies on a good understanding of what is happening.

New Zealand introduced new workplace health and safety legislation in 2015, to respond to major changes in the labour market and following the creation of WorkSafe as the country's primary health and safety regulator in 2013. Legislation, however, is still seen as safety oriented, enforcement in terms of work-related health is relatively poor and the capacity of the system to address psychosocial risks is not sufficient.

New Zealand is a role model with regard to mental health awareness campaigns that, more recently, also target the workplace as a priority setting. This, together with a range of toolkits prepared by Work Safe (e.g. bullying-prevention toolbox; guidelines on fatigue) but also the Mental Health Foundation and the Health Promotion Agency, has helped employers to understand the issue. Effective tools for employers are critical in a country in which workers can be dismissed relatively easily and at relatively short notice, in comparison with most other OECD countries.

New Zealand is providing limited assistance to employers facing reduced worker productivity resulting from mental health conditions, and mental health services are difficult to access for people who have a job. This is particularly challenging for the many small and micro businesses which lack the knowledge and resources to address problems or, at the very least, to contract an Employee Assistance Programme provider.

New Zealand has a unique Accident Compensation Corporation (ACC) system which provides comprehensive support in case of injury, work-related or not, on a no-fault basis. The success of the system, however, comes with considerable, undesirable side effects for illnesses, which do not receive the same attention. Stress-related illness and mental disorders in particular are outside the focus of ACC. Instead of investing resources in assessing claims and identifying cases that can be rejected, ACC's successful early intervention and rehabilitation approach should be adopted for illnesses as well to the extent possible – be it within an expanded ACC system or in other existing structures.

Prevention of psychosocial workplace risks should be strengthened

Employment is generally a positive factor for mental wellbeing and recovery from mental health conditions but high workplace stress and poor management can put a strain on mental health, exacerbate mental health conditions, and trigger the onset of a mental health condition. Employers' and workers' awareness of, and ability to identify and mitigate against, work environment risk factors potentially contributing to psychosocial harm is therefore critical. Failure to maintaining a healthy workforce will ultimately have detrimental effects for workers and businesses alike.

Working conditions are relatively good in New Zealand

New Zealand has a strong labour market. The overall employment rate, at 76.9% in 2017, is high, compared with the OECD average of 67.8%, and the unemployment rate, at 4.9% in 2017, is below the OECD average and gradually approaching pre-crisis levels (Figure 4.1). Long-term unemployment, at 15.6% of total unemployment in 2017, is half the OECD level. New Zealand's labour market is also quite inclusive: the employment gap for disadvantaged groups is lower in New Zealand than in the average OECD country. This is especially true for low-skilled and older workers but also workers with mental health problems (see Chapter 1). New Zealand is also doing relatively well in an OECD comparison of the quality of the work environment: just under one in four workers, 23.3% in 2015, are experiencing job strain. This is among the lowest values among countries for which comparable data are available, and significantly lower than the OECD average of 41%.

Figure 4.1. The labour market in New Zealand is strong and inclusive and working conditions are comparatively good

A scoreboard of labour market performance in terms of job quantity, job quality and inclusiveness

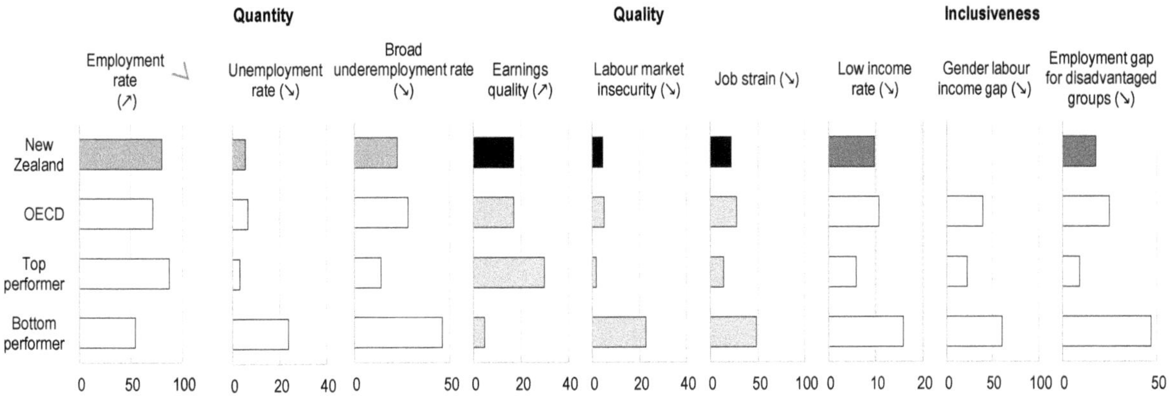

Note: An upward ↗ (downward ↘) pointing arrow for an indicator means that higher (lower) values reflect better performance.
Definitions: Broad underemployment: Share of inactive, unemployed or involuntary part-timers in population, excluding youth (15-29) in education and not in employment. *Earnings quality*: Gross hourly earnings in USD adjusted for inequality. *Labour market insecurity*: Expected monetary loss associated with becoming unemployed as a share of previous earnings. *Job strain*: Percentage of workers in jobs characterised by a combination of high job demands and few job resources to meet those demands. *Low income rate*: Share of working-age persons living with less than 50% of median equivalised household disposable income. *Gender labour income gap*: Difference between average per capita annual earnings of men and women divided by average per capita earnings of men. *Employment gap for disadvantaged groups*: Average difference in the employment rate for prime-age men and the rates for five disadvantaged groups (mothers with children, youth who are not in full-time education or training, workers aged 55-64, persons not born in the country, and persons with disabilities) as a percentage of the employment rate for prime-age men.
Source: OECD calculations using data for 2015 or latest year available from multiple sources. See OECD Employment Outlook 2017, http://dx.doi.org/10.1787/empl_outlook-2017-en, Table 1.2, http://dx.doi.org/10.1787/888933478165 for further details.

StatLink http://dx.doi.org/10.1787/888933845567

The latter is an encouraging finding, based on a unified methodology. However, it implies that one in four workers report job strain, a finding corroborated by national statistics based on the Survey of Working Life. In 2012, the last year for which data is available, 18.3% of workers in New Zealand found their work always or often stressful, and another 40% sometimes – irrespective of age and gender (Figure 4.2). Similarly, 13% say they are always or often too tired to enjoy life outside work, and another 31.5% sometimes. Finally, the survey shows that one in ten workers have experienced discrimination, harassment or bullying in the past 12 months (12.7% of women, 8.3% of men). Such figures suggest work puts strain on many people, also in New Zealand.[1]

Figure 4.2. Work can be stressful for many New Zealanders, at least sometimes

Perceived incidence in the past 12 months of various aspects of work-related health (percentage of workers)

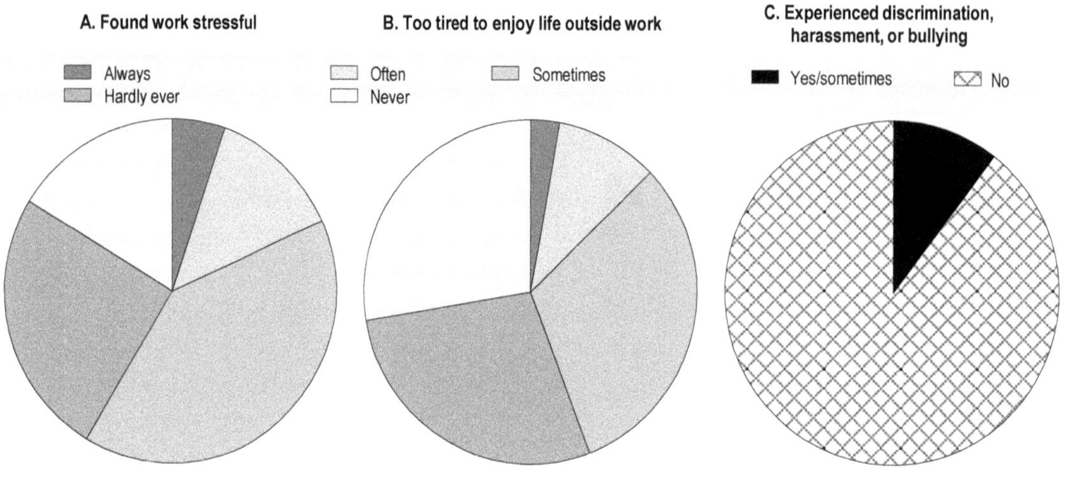

Source: Statistics New Zealand, Survey of Working Life: December 2012 quarter.

StatLink http://dx.doi.org/10.1787/888933845586

Little is known or published on the degree to which good working conditions are experienced evenly across the population – e.g. regionally or across ethnic groups. Earlier research has suggested Māori and Pacific Island populations experience more bullying but less psychological strain, maybe related to the better supervisor support they receive (Gardner et al., 2013[5]). Data from the Worker Exposure Survey confirm this finding: non-Māori report a higher prevalence of moderate stress (45% vs. 39% for Māori) and non-Māori men also a higher prevalence of extreme stress. Temporary employment, which generally offers poorer security and less protection, however, is more frequent among Māori (13%) compared with the rest of the population (8-9%).[2]

New workplace legislation has considerable potential

Statutory provisions for health and safety at work (including mental health) in New Zealand are addressed by the *Health and Safety at Work Act* of 2015, which came into force in April 2016. The Act replaced the former *Health and Safety in Employment Act*, from 1992, whose provisions were found to fail to guarantee health and safety (MBIE, 2013[6]; Independent Taskforce on Workplace Health and Safety, 2013[7]).

The new legislation introduced a number of key reforms to the previous system, guided by principles of participation, leadership, and accountability among government, employers and workers alike. The new legislation focuses on proactively anticipating and managing the underlying risks that might otherwise result in an injury or illness, in addition to monitoring and recording health and safety incidents. The reforms include a national target to reduce fatalities at work and serious work-related injuries by at least 25% by 2020 (Independent Taskforce on Workplace Health and Safety, 2013[8]).[3]

Workplace legislation covers all work-related health conditions; physical and psychological, acute and long-term. The Act requires the provision and maintenance of a work environment without risks to health and safety. In a special guide, WorkSafe provides a description of what that can mean; the psychological work environment can include "overcrowding, deadlines, work arrangements (e.g. the effects of shift-work and overtime arrangements), and impairments that affect a person's behaviour, such as work-related stress and fatigue, and drugs and alcohol" (WorkSafe, 2016[9]).

Where a work situation does result in a notifiable psychological injury, illness or incident, the Employment Relations Act provides a clear legal framework for liability and redress. The Ministry of Business, Innovation and Employment operates a free mediation service for employers and workers for some disputes, with 4 000-5 000 mediation cases per year of which 75% are resolved through the mediation procedure.

The 2015 Act is a step forward and addresses health in a broad sense. Its impact will depend on its enforcement. WorkSafe is working toward ensuring businesses are able to identify a range of risks and is developing a range of materials that will allow for intervention and the prevention of poor work-related health outcomes, including anxiety, depression and social isolation, possibly as a result of physical health hazards. In implementing the objectives of the Act, looking at other countries can be useful. In Belgium, for example, in addition to preparing a psychosocial risk analysis, employers are required to draw up a global five-year prevention plan and more concrete annual action plans. They also have to appoint a psychosocial prevention advisor to assist them in implementing the risk prevention plan (OECD, 2013[10]).

WorkSafe is moving into its broader role

In late 2013, a new crown entity was established, WorkSafe New Zealand, as the country's prime workplace health and safety regulator.[4] WorkSafe's mandate was further clarified under the Health and Safety at Work Act in 2015, to include three distinct roles: First, regulating workplaces to ensure they manage health and safety appropriately. Second, preventing harm by targeting critical risks at various levels, influencing attitudes and behaviour and intervening, where necessary. Third, providing broader leadership over the health and safety system to improve work-related health and safety outcomes.

WorkSafe has developed three strategic documents to help guide its activities into the mid-2020s:

- A Strategic Plan for Work-Related Health 2016-26, outlining its approach to achieving "improved awareness, attitudes and behaviours around work-related health and, through these, better management of work-related health risks and reduced exposures to health hazards" (WorkSafe, 2016[11]). The strategy explicitly recognises psychosocial risks as one of five key categories of work-related health risks (alongside physical, chemical, biological and ergonomic risks) and includes these as a priority for targeted programmes.
- A joint action plan to reduce harm in workplaces for the period 2016-26, in partnership with ACC (WorkSafe and ACC, 2016[12]). Due to the mandate of ACC (see more below), the plan almost exclusively focuses on physical health.
- A formal strategy for improving workplace health and safety for Māori called Maruiti 2025 (derived from the Māori concept of a safe haven). Among its outcomes, the strategy aims to lower workplace injuries, health-related incidents and fatalities in the Māori community to the levels of the non-Māori population by the year 2025. However, the strategy does not explicitly address work-related mental harm and associated risks.

An independent review was completed in late 2015 that applauded WorkSafe for its high performance at a relatively early stage of development (Martin, 2015[13]). The review made several recommendations some of which WorkSafe has since taken up but it did not choose to focus in any depth or detail on WorkSafe's newer role around the psychological aspects of workplace health and safety. WorkSafe is gradually shifting its focus to its wider role, including educating employers, within its existing resources. At this stage, WorkSafe has no specific targets on reducing psychosocial risks or on the implementation of risk prevention plans by employers and, similar to the situation in other OECD countries, its inspectors generally lack psychosocial expertise. As society's expectations change, WorkSafe's capability and capacity would need to change alongside and additional resources would be required to deliver on those expectations.

Strengthening the implementation of workplace health and safety

WorkSafe appears to have a large and active role around physical safety. By comparison, however, WorkSafe's coverage of mental health and of psychosocial risks to health still appears to be rather weak. WorkSafe has a clear mandate for this under the new *Health and Safety at Work Act*. Considerably more can be done in this space, in terms of prevention of harm and provision of leadership, to reduce the number of workers facing psychosocial risks and seeing their mental health deteriorate. WorkSafe is growing its maturity of thinking in this area which has the added complexity of non-work factors contributing to, or exacerbating, workers' poor psychological health.

One key challenge for WorkSafe is the collection of better data. Today, WorkSafe relies heavily on ACC data, which largely include physical injury harm. To become a modern intelligence-led regulator would require significant investment in data collection (including statistics by ethnicity, gender and age to identify particular risk groups and corresponding risk-prevention strategies) and corresponding IT systems.

Dealing with cases of work-related mental distress or harassment places high demands on employers, workers and WorkSafe. WorkSafe has limited resources and is therefore only able to investigate the most serious cases of work-related harm. Investigation and enforcement activities are risk-based and targeted at the highest risks and harm. In line with this, cases of work-related mental distress or bullying carry a high burden of evidence for workers – including a formal diagnosis from a mental health professional and a paper trail of the abusive behaviour they have been subjected to – before WorkSafe can launch an investigation. Workers also must observe a 90-day notification period since the incident occurred to be able to access any services (beyond this period, they would have to meet the threshold of a serious crime that was investigated by the police). The result of these limitations is that WorkSafe has reportedly investigated only 13 complaints of workplace bullying out of 159 total bullying concerns notified to it since its establishment in late 2013. When notifications do not meet WorkSafe's criteria for an investigation, people are provided with assistance through referral to another appropriate organisation or to WorkSafe's guidance resources on workplace bullying.

WorkSafe's role goes further than investigating mental health complaints and includes supporting employers in their effort to identify and prevent psychosocial risks. For this to happen more systematically, inspectors will need much better competence on mental health and psychosocial risks and WorkSafe would need additional funding to recruit technical experts in work-related psychosocial matters. To promote this, WorkSafe could set itself two targets every year, one related to reducing physical health risks and one to preventing psychosocial workplace risks and stressors.

Moving forward in better enforcing its health and safety legislation, New Zealand can perhaps adopt some of the approaches used in other OECD countries. Denmark provides an interesting example for how to support employers in their new role. The Danish Working Environment Authority has developed a series of 24 both sector- and job-specific guidance tools which describe the prevalence of risk factors and the potential resources a company has to prevent psychosocial problems (OECD, 2013[14]). Inspectors have been trained in how to use these guidance tools, and there are a smaller number of expert inspectors who can assist other inspectors in assessing psychosocial workplace risks and in preparing improvement notices. This goes beyond WorkSafe's guidance on bullying prevention the purpose of which is also to support its frontline inspectors who also undergo basic module-based training on a number of psychosocial issues in the workplace. Resources in the bullying prevention toolbox are aimed specifically at small businesses and at workers.[5]

The time might now be right for a renewed focus on the psychological aspects of workplace health and safety. Representatives of New Zealand employers' organisations report a sense of increased responsibility and "ownership" around ensuring workers' mental health and generating the necessary dialogue around what individuals might be experiencing. In Canterbury, in particular, the earthquakes that have happened since 2011 have put significant pressure on people's mental health (Fergusson et al., 2014[15]) and, in effect, produced a catalyst for better engagement around mental health and reduced some of the previous stigma and misunderstanding (Calder et al., 2016[16]).[6]

Addressing stigma, discrimination and misconceptions

Because mental health conditions are so prevalent in the working-age population, most workplaces will be affected to some degree or at some stage and have to address the resulting consequences. Nevertheless, stigmatising environments towards mental health conditions continue to persist in many workplaces and often make matters worse for those experiencing them. Discrimination may also be common. Such dynamic may discourage workers from disclosing a mental health concern, in turn further increasing stigma and enforcing misconceptions. The dynamics can also create self-stigma, which reduces individuals' feeling of self-worth, isolating them further and delaying help-seeking and, thereby, impeding their recovery (Thornicroft et al., 2016[17]).

The *Human Rights Act*, from 1993, prohibits discrimination on the grounds of disability. Under a broad definition, this includes (among others): "(iii) Psychiatric illness; (iv) Intellectual or psychological disability or impairment; and (v) Any other loss or abnormality of psychological, physiological, or anatomical structure or function". The United Nations *Convention on the Rights of Persons with Disabilities*, from 2006, likewise applies to individuals with "mental and intellectual impairments" and contains prescriptions around work and employment-related discrimination.

A number of public and non-governmental organisations in New Zealand operate initiatives and campaigns combatting stigma, discrimination and misconceptions around mental health in workplaces. Over time, this has increased awareness of the issues among the general population considerably. Only more recently, however, have these campaigns included a focus on work and employment; this is a very important shift in focus, which should be built upon.

Anti-stigma campaigns and toolkits for employers are plentiful

The Mental Health Foundation is a prominent organisation combatting mental health-related stigma in New Zealand. At the forefront of its work on reducing workplace stigma is the *Open Minds* campaign, which promotes an online collection of information and training materials aimed at equipping business leaders with the tools and confidence to engage with their workers around potential issues to do with mental health (Mental Health Foundation, 2017[18]). The Mental Health Foundation's *Five Ways to Wellbeing at Work Toolkit* (Mental Health Foundation and Health Promotion Agency, 2018[19]) and its *Working Well* resources (Mental Health Foundation, 2016[20]) also offer additional guidance for employers and examples of good conduct in this area. The Mental Health Foundation also partners with other organisations for the online space *Wellplace.nz* where employers can access useful tips and tools for building healthier workplaces.[7]

Another organisation doing prominent work in this area is the Health Promotion Agency, which, most importantly, heads *Like Minds, Like Mine* – New Zealand's longest-running campaign combatting stigma around mental health (established in 1997). The stated goal of the campaign is to achieve respectful attitudes and inclusive behaviours towards individuals with experience of mental illness and distress (see also Chapter 2). In its latest version, Like Minds, Like Mine has emphasised the role of employment as a key to recovery. One of the forthcoming three-year community initiatives will have an explicit focus on workplaces and employers, because of an increasing number of requests on behalf of employers in response to the new *Health and Safety at Work Act*.

The Health Promotion Agency also partners with other organisations to host an interactive online tool called *Good4Work* that enterprises can use to access useful advice and information (similar to what *Wellspace.nz* offers).

The Ministry of Social Development (MSD) operates a free telephone line under its *Disability Confident* campaign that business leaders and managers can call to gain advice around supporting or managing a worker with a disability or health condition, including mental health conditions. More recently, all kinds of helplines for employers as well as persons with health problems or addiction were brought under the umbrella of a new National Telehealth Service, including the Employer Advice Line. The staff that administer the Employer Advice Line are health advisors employed by Homecare Medical, which is contracted by MSD to deliver the service.

Raising awareness and combatting misinformation

Despite a range of available tools, employers in New Zealand reportedly seldom know where to turn or what support they might get when a worker encounters trouble with their mental health. This is partly explained by the disconnect between programmes and resources for managing mental health at work (i.e. employment relationships, public health, human rights, or workplace health and safety). Many employers may fail to engage with the resources on offer before the issue develops into a more significant mental health crisis for the worker and, in turn, the company. In the worst case, employers' actions may instead fuel the fire if dictated by misconceptions by, for example, piling social or professional pressure onto an underperforming worker or neglecting early warning signs.

However, the private sector is also more and more active in this field.[8] As in other OECD countries, some large companies in New Zealand are leading this development, driven by strong leadership. Air New Zealand, Bank of New Zealand, Fonterra, Z-Energy and

Vodafone are the ones mentioned most frequently in this context. But the bigger challenge is to involve also smaller and medium-sized businesses which, similar to other countries, make up 95% of New Zealand's companies and employ half of the New Zealand workforce.[9]

Some companies in New Zealand have recently moved to create positions for health and wellbeing managers within their human resources departments. A group of such businesses – both large and small – recently came together to form a community of such professionals under the Business Leaders' Health and Safety Forum and through the *Health and Wellbeing Leaders' Network* to develop leadership and share examples of best practices. Their priority themes for 2017 included: building relationships with government agencies such as WorkSafe and ACC; empowering health and wellbeing professionals in their companies; and building media presence to reach out to a larger number of stakeholders.

The driving forces behind this network are *Fonterra* (a dairy nutrition company employing 22 000 people globally and 11 500 in New Zealand) and *Z-energy* (a fuel distributor with branded service stations and around 3 000 employees). Both of these companies have strong health and wellbeing policies in place, with a reported return on investment in the order of 2.3 dollars for every dollar put in. Their company policies have a strong focus on resilience and training for managers, annual health surveillance, immediate intervention (including by a clinical psychologist) and peer-to-peer support.

Equipping employers with the knowledge to address such issues in a timely way could be a valuable starting point towards managing psychological risks properly. Employers clearly have an important role to play in complementing social, family and whānau networks. Numerous common life-events represent times when workers may feel exacerbated pressures around their mental health. Such events may also be sector- or business-specific including droughts (for farmers), competitive pressures (for manufacturers and others), technological change (especially for medium-skill industries) and business downturns or periods of retrenchment, more generally. Such events are generally knowable to supervisors and can act as potential red flags to increase vigilance and engage in active dialogue and support, if needed. Left unchecked, or unsupported, such common pressures can manifest into diagnosable mental health conditions.

In conclusion, it appears that there is no lack in New Zealand of campaigns and support tools for employers. The recent inclusion in the various campaigns of a work and workplace focus should be continued and its impact measured. For the support tools, the biggest challenge is dissemination to ensure a wide use by employers. This requires the involvement of private actors and networks with good access to employers. Evaluating the various support tools and their impact in the workplace is important; also as a way to market successful tools to employers.

Understanding the link between mental health and productivity

Mental health conditions can be very costly for employers. Workers experiencing such conditions are absent from work more frequently, on average, and spend longer periods off work than workers with other health concerns. However, the loss in labour productivity is even larger. Workers who experience mental health conditions report performance-related problems more often than others; workers with active symptoms of mild-to-moderate mental health conditions in particular would typically not take extra sick leave but show considerable underperformance while in work if their symptoms remain unrecognised, untreated and unsupported, potentially also affecting their co-workers (OECD, 2015[1]). These dynamics affect the performance of every business.

Evidence on absenteeism and presenteeism is lacking

Unlike most other OECD countries, New Zealand does not routinely collect data on sickness absence. Knowledge about the extent of the problem absenteeism presents for businesses, relevant trends over time, and underlying reasons underpinning sickness absences is therefore limited. This represents an important omission under the current labour market information system and a crucial knowledge gap for policy makers.

Most OECD countries gather data on sickness absences in a systematic manner in two ways. First, virtually all countries collect self-reported information on absence in their regular labour force surveys. Such information, by definition, includes short as well as long-term absences and is therefore the best source for comparative statistics. As is commonly known, however, subjective data will underreport the true level of absence. Secondly, a subset of countries with statutory cash sickness benefits also collect information of absences lasting longer than a certain threshold (i.e. those which generate insurance or benefit entitlements) through their administrative sickness benefit statistics (Vester Thorsen et al., 2015[21]). Such data are more reliable and more detailed (e.g. by duration of absence) but less comparable across countries because of different thresholds used and the large difference in the functioning of the benefit system.

New Zealand is not collecting any self-reported absence data through any of its population surveys and does not have comparable administrative statistics because it does not have a statutory cash sickness benefit. The only data available in New Zealand related to sickness at least to a certain degree are statistics on jobseeker benefit recipients with a health or disability designation (discussed in more detail in Chapter 5). Due to the nature of the benefit payments, which are means-tested and paid to those out of work, however, these numbers do not present any even remote estimate of the level of employee sickness absence in New Zealand.

The only rough information available on sickness absence in New Zealand comes from the *Wellness in the Workplace* survey; a survey run every two years and sponsored by Business New Zealand, jointly with the Southern Cross Health Society. It is a survey answered by employers who are asked about the average number of days of absence of their employees.[10] In 2016, the overall absence was 4.4 days per employee, which is a very low figure in international comparison. Absence levels are higher in the public than in the private sector; higher among manual than non-manual workers; and higher in larger than in smaller companies. Employer-identified absence rates have remained rather stable over time (4.7 days per employee in 2014 and 4.5 days in 2012).

The main drivers of absence in New Zealand were non-work-related illnesses (typically minor illnesses) followed by caring for a sick family member and non-work-related injuries, together explaining more than two-thirds of all sickness absences. Work-related injury and illness plays a minor role. Anxiety, stress and depression is much more prevalent as a cause of absence for non-manual workers but non-work-related anxiety, stress and depression also plays an increasing role for manual workers (BusinessNZ and Southern Cross Health Society, 2017[2]).

There is strong reason to believe that the relatively low level of sickness absence is related to New Zealand's limited sick pay regulations (see below). As a consequence, presenteeism – people turning up for work even though they should stay home due to illness – is likely to be high. The full extent of presenteeism is unknown but the same employer survey also contains hints about the degree to which employees come to work sick: some four in five employees commonly seem to do so, according to their employers' impression, with only one in five rarely or almost never coming to work sick. As expected, presenteeism is more common in the private sector in New Zealand. On the other hand, the survey also suggests that the large majority of businesses have a culture of encouraging employees to remain away from work if they are ill.

It is disturbing that New Zealand has never made an effort to collect data on employee sickness absence in a more systematic manner. Such information is critical for policy makers in understanding the impact of existing rules. Every effort should be made to include questions that are used in other OECD countries in several of New Zealand's population surveys, including especially the Labour Force Survey and the New Zealand Health Survey.

Employer-provided sick leave is meagre

In New Zealand, sickness is a topic that does not get the attention it deserves, in terms of data but also corresponding policies. Consequently, there is only limited protection available for workers falling ill. Under New Zealand's *Holidays Act*, from 2003, most employees are entitled to 5-20 days of paid sick leave on a statutory basis.[11] Within the first six months of their work, a new employee is not entitled to any paid leave under the statutory rules. Beyond the first six months, however, employees gain statutory rights to five days of paid sickness absence per year, with the ability to carry over unspent days up to a maximum allowance of 20 days at any given point in time. When paid sick days are used up workers can use their annual leave entitlement instead or seek unpaid sick leave.[12]

Nothing is known about the actual sick-pay entitlements workers in New Zealand can access and for how long. Data from the 2012 Survey of Working Life give some hints in this regard although the information available is about *total* paid leave entitlements, not sick leave entitlements. Permanent workers, a group comprising 90% of all employees in New Zealand, typically have four weeks of paid leave every year, with a significant minority of 18% having more than four weeks and a minority of almost 8% having no such entitlement; half of the latter will instead have a slightly higher wage (Figure 4.3). The situation is very different for casual workers who rarely have any leave entitlements. Half of them, however, will have casual loading i.e. a somewhat higher wage that compensates the lacking leave entitlement. Temporary workers will find all kinds of situations although also among them one in four have no leave entitlements. This suggests that not having any sick pay in case of an illness is a common situation for temporary and especially casual workers. Permanent workers will have some entitlements but they rarely seem to go beyond the statutory minimum.

From an international perspective, it is surprising how little discussion there is in New Zealand about the poor protection of workers falling ill. Only two other OECD countries, Korea and the United States, find themselves in a similar situation, partly explaining high levels of poverty in all three countries for this group of people. Research in the United States has repeatedly shown that the lack of sick-pay in most States leads to higher rates of presenteeism for seriously ill people who should stay home, thereby increasing infection of co-workers (Drago and Miller, 2010$_{[22]}$). Likewise, research has demonstrated that paid sick days benefit both the employer e.g. in the form of reduced turnover and work injuries and the worker e.g. through improved employment stability, higher labour force attachment and more timely treatment (Milli, Xia and Min, 2016[23]). There is considerable room for New Zealand to improve the situation, by extending the period of employer liability and broadening entitlements for non-permanent workers.

Figure 4.3. Permanent employees in New Zealand are entitled to four weeks of paid leave

Distribution of New Zealand employees by type of work contract and annual entitlement to paid leave

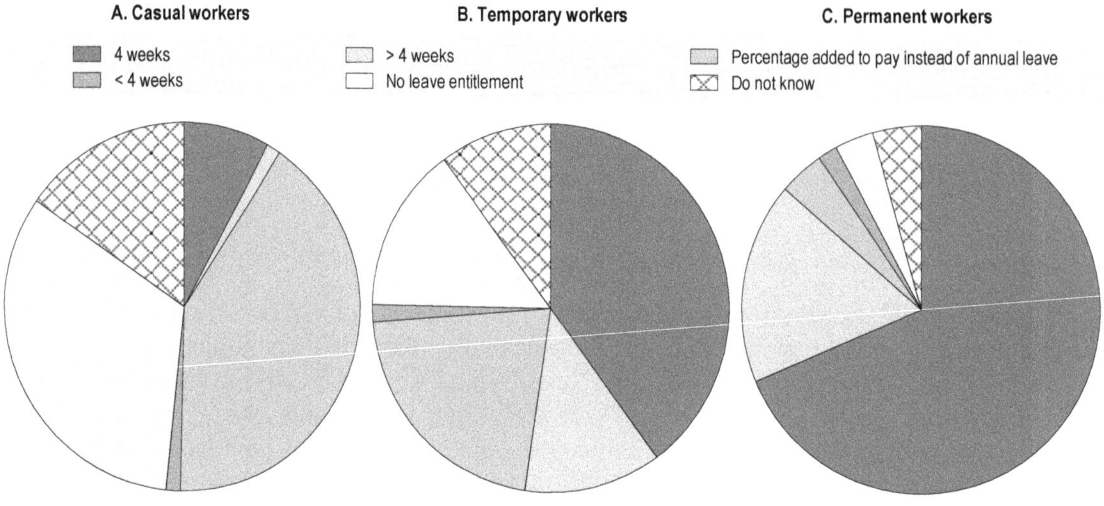

Note: Of all employees in New Zealand in 2012, 89% were permanent workers. Another 5% were casual workers, 4% fixed-term or temporary agency workers, and the remainder seasonal workers.
Source: Statistics New Zealand, Survey of Working Life: December 2012 quarter.

StatLink http://dx.doi.org/10.1787/888933845605

Protection for sickness is much broader in other OECD countries

Most OECD countries implement income support measures for employees undergoing temporary absences from work related to illness or injury. Countries typically use a combination of two types of policy measures:

- *Employer liability for sickness* places a burden of duty on employers to provide for eligible workers during a period of ill health. Employers may be obliged to pay part (or all) their worker's salary, over a specified period of their absence.
- *Cash sickness benefits* can provide more extensive income support for workers in case of sickness beyond the period of employer liability. Such income support could be related to the worker's own earnings but it could also be means-tested.

Many OECD countries mandate employers to continue paying an absent worker (in full or in part) over a period of around one to three working weeks. In several cases, however, employer liability covers a much longer potential period of time: extending to around six weeks in Germany and Poland; 11-12 weeks in Austria and Luxembourg; 18 weeks for some workers in France; 26 weeks in the United Kingdom; 36 weeks in Italy; and two years in the Netherlands (Spasova, Bouget and Vanhercke, 2016[24]). In some countries, such as Switzerland, Israel, Finland and France, employers may be bound to equivalent obligations under the terms of their workers' employment contracts or via a collective agreement. In countries that do not regulate employer liability, such as Canada and the United States, it is predominantly at employers' own discretion to decide what support to offer a sick worker.

Cash sickness benefits usually extend far beyond the limited provisions of employer liability for sickness. Korea and the United States, together with New Zealand, are the only OECD countries which do not have a dedicated cash sickness benefit programme.

Figure 4.4 illustrates the income protection provided to employees for sickness in selected OECD countries. Three dimensions determine the scope of income support, which cash sickness benefits may provide: the maximum *duration* for which cash sickness benefits are paid; the *value* of the cash income support provided; and the *interaction between cash sickness benefits and employer liability*.

First, some countries offer support for relatively limited periods of time (such as 15 weeks in Canada) while others do so for up to 18 months or longer (such as Germany, the Netherlands, Portugal or Japan) or indefinite periods of time in case a recovery is expected (such as in Slovenia and the United Kingdom) (Social Security Administration, 2016[25]). Secondly, most cash sickness benefits are calculated as a share of the claimants' usual work-related income, commonly compensating anything from 50% of this amount (as in Canada) to 70% in most countries (including Germany, Portugal, Japan and the Netherlands) to all of it (as in Luxembourg and in some of the Nordic countries), subject to floor and ceiling amounts. Thirdly, some countries rely exclusively on employers' liability (such as the Netherlands and Switzerland) while others have only social insurance without any employer liability (such as Canada, Japan or Portugal). Most, however, rely to some extent on both (Spasova, Bouget and Vanhercke, 2016[24]). In some countries, such as Portugal, sickness compensation varies over time while in others, such as Luxembourg, employers pool their own liability risks through a mutual insurance fund. Such collective insurance can be operated nationally or privately. Mandatory schemes also sometimes entail opt-out clauses for large firms that are big enough to manage their own risks unilaterally.

The six cases outlined in Figure 4.4 illustrate a variety of possible approaches to providing social protection for sickness, although they are not exhaustive. The majority of OECD countries provide cash sickness benefits for a period of at least six months, in accordance with medical evidence on treatment and recovery times which suggests that such length of leave is important to cover more severe illnesses (Raub et al., 2018[26]). Most systems also replace a large part of a worker's wage to prevent harsh income losses. As the social protection system in New Zealand is entirely means-tested, providing cash support only to those in acute need, introducing a significant degree of statutory liability for employers for all workers who fall sick – beyond current limited sick-leave entitlements – would seem an important step to take. This would strongly increase the incentives for employers to attend to psychosocial workplace risks, and their responsiveness to mental health issues in the workplace (Kendall et al., 2015[27]).

Like in other OECD countries, insurance companies in New Zealand also offer private income protection insurance for people temporarily ill. Because of the lack of a publicly or privately regulated sickness cash benefit programme, such private insurance plays a more critical role in New Zealand than in other countries where such insurance will often just top-up public entitlements. Little is known about insurance coverage and the type of protection offered in New Zealand. Estimates from the insurance sector suggest that some 17-20% of the workforce has access to private income protection insurance (Financial Services Council, 2017[28]). Insurance can be individual or group based and will involve risk-rated premiums. The extent to which these premiums are covered by employers and/or employees is unknown. The scope and level of support can differ considerably between insurance products: ranging from income protection for several months or a year (i.e. like other countries' cash sickness benefit payments), to the entire working life until age 65 (i.e. like a generous disability insurance payment).

Figure 4.4. OECD countries offer very different levels of income support for sickness

Maximum duration, value and type of income support for sickness in selected OECD countries, 2016

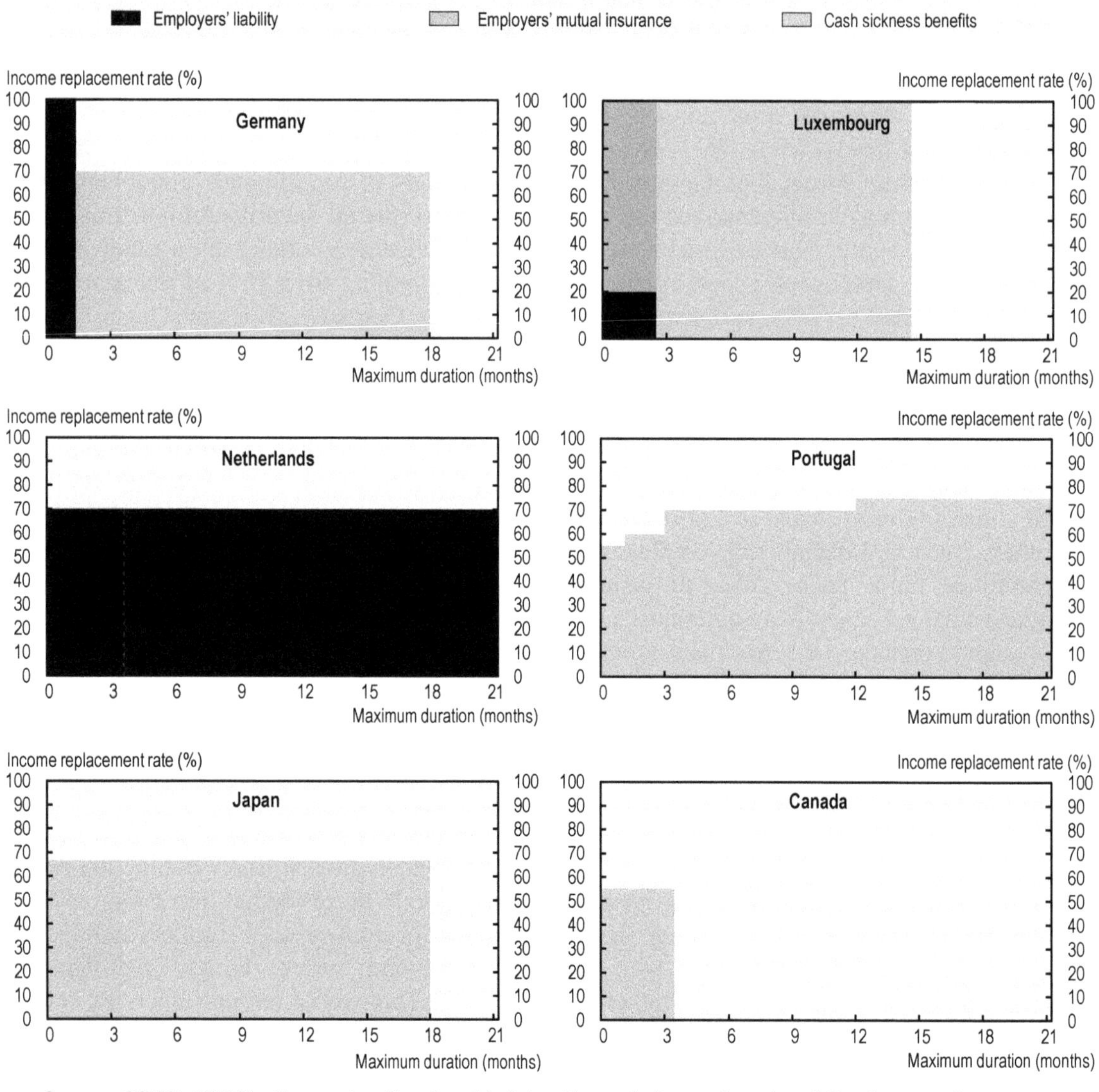

Source: OECD (2018), *Connecting People with Jobs: Towards Better Social and Employment Security in Korea*, OECD Publishing, Paris.

StatLink http://dx.doi.org/10.1787/888933845624

Overall, the minimal available evidence suggests that only few New Zealanders have private income protection insurance, with considerable differences across insurance contracts. It is also likely that within-company inequity is considerable. There are no data available to corroborate this but similar data on private health insurance coverage offered by New Zealand companies show that of all those companies which offer such insurance, only around 60% do so for all of their employees (BusinessNZ and Southern Cross Health Society, 2017[2]). These data also show that large companies are much more likely to offer private health insurance: coverage rates range from 16% in companies with less than 50 employees to over 60% in companies with 50 or more employees (the overall average is around 40%). While this suggests that private health insurance is more common in New Zealand businesses than private income protection insurance, it is likely that coverage rate differences are similar. An alternative strategy for New Zealand therefore could be to promote income protection insurance, for example through tax deductions for insurance premiums especially for small and medium-sized companies, with the aim to reduce workforce inequalities.

Managing workplace stress and mental health problems

With limited income support available for workers who are ill and temporarily unable to work, compared with other OECD countries, coupled with lenient employment protection legislation in comparison with the OECD average (OECD, 2013[29]), there is a considerable risk in New Zealand, higher than in other OECD countries, that sick workers could lose their job. This raises questions about workplace practices in New Zealand to monitor sickness absence and about the support that is available to manage workplace stress and mental health problems of workers and to prevent presenteeism and absenteeism.

Employee Assistance Programmes (EAPs) appear to be the principal stay-at-work support available for workers encountering mental health difficulties in New Zealand. Companies often offer EAPs to their employees as part of their wider health and safety programme or as part of a broader managing-diversity strategy. The 2017 Wellness in the Workplace Survey indicates that four in five large companies in New Zealand, with 50 and more employees, contract an EAP provider. Among smaller companies, which represent 43% of the labour market, however, the corresponding share is only around 30%. Smaller firms are also less commonly offering the possibility to work from home or more flexible hours, as a way to accommodate personal circumstances.

EAPs give employers the ability to pay someone else to take a problem off their hands. They offer confidential, short-term counselling for employees with personal problems that affect their work performance, whether or not those problems originate in the workplace. The exact set of supports will vary from provider to provider, as there are no regulations in place in New Zealand on minimal support an EAP provider must offer. There are different options for organisations to provide EAP to staff including:

- Contracting a single provider and paying a set fee based on the number of workers in the organisation. Such the employer does not know who is using the service so employees can feel that their use of the service is completely confidential.
- Contracting a single provider and paying per counselling session. This can be done more confidentially if the employee can go through a designated contact person in the organisation, so the person's name can be protected.
- Contracting with specific providers as and when needed. The advantage of this is that specialist providers can be used, targeting the person's specific situation. Again, if a designated contact person is available within the organisation, this will assist with the protection of the person's name.

EAPs provide a useful mediator for complex situations, including bullying and abuse cases, typically including three counselling sessions free of charge though some employers may go beyond and pay for more tailored psychological support. One of the problems is that EAPs generally provide little guidance for employers to understand the problems and their relationship to the workplace. Confidentiality can force employers into a situation where they do not know what is going on with an employee or how best to facilitate their recovery.

Nevertheless, EAPs are a useful tool and efforts should be made in New Zealand to increase coverage in small and medium-sized firms, which tend to be less aware of the need for action. For example, while larger companies make various efforts to identify workplace stress through staff surveys or the provision of training to managers to identify and manage stress, this is rarely the case in smaller companies (BusinessNZ and Southern Cross Health Society, 2017[2]). Research in the United States has shown that contracting an EAP provider can contribute to decreased absenteeism, greater employee retention and reduced medical costs because of earlier treatment (Hargrave et al., 2008[30]; Lam and Walker, 2012[31]). Contracting EAP providers should be facilitated and could be supported financially for smaller companies, and minimum standards should be regulated to ensure all EAP providers offer a basic set of supports.

However, EAPs alone will not be enough; other structures and systems need to be improved or involved. For instance, New Zealand's employment service, Work and Income, will not intervene until a person has actually lost their job and entered onto benefits. In other countries, the Public Employment Service or the Social Insurance Authority has a strong role in dealing with health-related problems in the workplace early on. In Norway, for example, every employer has a contact person in the local labour and welfare office who can provide advice and refer employers or employees quickly to the right service (OECD, 2013[32]). In Switzerland, as another example, the disability insurance authority has invested considerably in helping employers quickly when health-related problems arise – in order to prevent much larger costs for them later for people dropping out of the labour market altogether (OECD, 2014[33]).

More generally, occupational health knowledge in workplaces is of paramount importance in the light of the fact that good work contributes to good health and good health improves engagement and performance. Several OECD countries have strong occupational health policies in place encouraging employers to bring corresponding knowledge into their company. In the Netherlands, for example, occupational physicians are a part of company life, as the law obliges employers to consult an occupational physician in managing their workers' sicknesses (OECD, 2014[34]).

Statutory regulations are limited. New Zealand's *Employment Relations Act* ensures employees have a right to request alternative working arrangements from their employer in relation to their working hours, working days and place of work. This provision encourages employers and employees to have an open discussion on how to manage work-life and balance it against any external factors; this could contribute to reduced absenteeism, increased employee engagement and improved productivity. While employers are obliged to deal as quickly as possible with request for alternative working arrangements, they may also refuse to accommodate them on a variety of grounds. However, New Zealand's *Human Rights Act* and the *Health and Safety at Work Act* not only oblige employers to manage workplace hazards – including those applicable to mental health – but also to implement reasonable accommodations to address particular needs, where necessary. In some cases, such an accommodation may include a gradual return to work.

There is ongoing work to ensure all employees and employers understand their employment rights and obligations. The work includes pre-employment guides that assist employers and recruiters in complying with anti-discrimination provisions under the Human Rights Act and the Flexible Working Policy Builder, an online tool to help employers develop workplace policies on flexible work arrangements. In mid-2018, Business NZ launched a new health and wellbeing policy as part of the Workplace Policy Builder, a tool that allows businesses to create a variety of policies tailored to the needs of their workplace, covering a range of health and wellbeing-related topics.

Ultimately, the biggest challenge is to support smaller and medium-sized enterprises in their efforts to help employees with stress and mental health-related problems. Larger companies can invest in a broader health and wellbeing strategy, which may include private income protection as well as health insurance and a support plan that involves the employee, the manager and a health professional such as a mental health nurse. Smaller companies rely on structures that they can access and afford.

Improving return-to-work policies and processes

When workers fall ill and stop working, initially for a temporary period, providing cash benefits is only one aspect. Protection for sickness also requires a sound strategy for rehabilitation and return-to-work to ensure workers return to work quickly and with re-established work capacity. Such strategies seek to reintegrate beneficiaries in their former workplace or, if they have lost their job in the meantime, into the labour market more generally. It is of utmost importance to avoid longer sickness absences from work. Data for the United Kingdom show that four weeks of sickness absence is a critical intervention point (Black and Frost, 2011[35]) and data for a number of other OECD countries show that after three months of absence, the likelihood of a return to the labour market is very low (OECD, 2015[1]). Return-to-work strategies are also fundamental for combatting benefit traps cash sickness benefits may encounter – something that is hardly an issue in New Zealand, however, unless people have access to private income protection insurance.

Return-to-work strategies in OECD countries are diverse

A comprehensive return-to-work strategy is particularly important for workers on sick leave on the grounds of mental health conditions. For many mental health problems, the alienation from work can lead to an alienation from society thus exacerbating the health problem. As work generally contributes to recovery, being on sick leave for a longer period can be counterproductive. At the same time, for some workers work will often have contributed to their mental health problems, thereby making a return to the previous job less attractive.

OECD countries approach rehabilitation and return-to-work in a variety of ways. For example, some countries (like Austria, Denmark or Finland) provide partial capacity benefits for beneficiaries returning to work gradually upon regaining their work capacity (Spasova, Bouget and Vanhercke, 2016[24]). Research from Finland, which has introduced such legislation only recently, shows that a gradual return to work helps people to achieve higher rates of work participation (Kausto et al., 2014[36]). Some OECD countries build rehabilitation conditions into the entitlement rules of their benefit measures. Sickness benefits in Sweden, for example, apply a "rehabilitation chain" to ensure beneficiaries regain employment if they can. In the first 90 days, the aim is to return the worker into the previous job; in the next 90 days into any other job for the same employer; and thereafter into any job in the Swedish labour market (OECD, 2013[37]). Beneficiaries undergo a medical assessment at each stage in the chain to determine their work capacity. Other countries provide rehabilitation through the supporting services they provide under their health service, their public employment service or, possibly, some entity specialised in dealing with helping workers on sick leave. The United Kingdom, for example, launched its *Fit for Work* service in 2015, after a trial phase of several years, to provide advice and case-managed rehabilitation and return-to-work support, via telephone or online, to employers, employees and general practitioners. The optional service is free to access after four weeks of sick leave. Similar services operate in other OECD countries, e.g. Austria, Ireland or the Netherlands, where sometimes quick referral to psychological therapy is also possible (OECD, 2014[38]; Department for Work and Pensions, 2015[39]).

In New Zealand, little is in place for workers who are sick unless they or their employer has purchased income protection insurance. The latter contracts will often include early capacity assessment, rehabilitation and access to psychological therapy, especially if the insurance product contains longer-term benefit payments – largely for economic reasons to contain the costs arising from potentially long insurance claims.

Otherwise, return to work after a sickness absence is a highly under-recognised issue in policies and workplace practices in New Zealand. In this regard, a new initiative jointly started by the New Zealand Chamber of Commerce and Pegasus Health, a primary health organisation, is worth mentioning as it aims to increase the awareness of the issue among employers and doctors and to bring employers and doctors together in an effort to return employees on sick leave back to work faster. It will be important to follow this initiative closely and evaluate it rigorously and to explore its potential for a broader scale-up.

ACC is slowly recognising mental injury claims

One public system in New Zealand, nevertheless, has a strong focus on early intervention, medical and occupational assessment, vocational rehabilitation, and a fast return to work: the Accident Compensation Corporation system (ACC). ACC however, only covers accidents and related injuries, not illnesses unless they are caused by work. Injuries are covered on a no-blame basis irrespective of whether they are work-related.

Since October 2008, ACC also provides compensation for "work-related mental injuries" involving a discrete causative event at work resulting in a clinically significant behavioural, cognitive or psychological dysfunction.[13] ACC requires successful claims for work-related mental injury to meet a number of criteria (ACC, 2018[40]):

- The injury was caused by a discrete event that occurred suddenly (i.e. arose quickly with little or no warning).
- The causal event occurred in a person's place of employment or has a direct causal link to their work.
- The person must be in employment, defined as "work for the purpose of pecuniary gain or profit", thus excluding volunteer work.14
- The claimant has a diagnosed behavioural, cognitive or psychological dysfunction (temporary distress that constitutes a normal reaction to trauma is not covered).
- The event must reasonably be expected to cause mental injury to people generally (i.e. it would provoke extreme distress, horror or alarm in almost everyone and it falls outside the normal range of human experience).

ACC can thus provide compensation for workers exposed to a traumatic event within the workplace but not for those developing mental health conditions via gradual, cumulative or chronic work-related stressors or events that reoccur over a sustained period, such as workplace bullying. Thus, the potentially entitled group is small with less than 100 such claims every year. The share of mental injury claims in total ACC claims fluctuates around 0.1% or 1 500-2 000 claims every year, out of 1.9 million total claims.[15] The unentitled group contains the large majority of those experiencing problems around mental health since mental health conditions are considerably more prevalent than the mental injuries under ACC's narrow definition.

Return-to-work support under ACC can be comprehensive

For coverable conditions, ACC may provide occupational therapy and coordinate with a claimant's employer as part of a gradual return-to-work or rehabilitation plan. Vocational rehabilitation is open to individuals who are currently employed but absent from their work or not employed but encountering a loss of *potential* earnings (including students, for example, and unemployed persons).

For recognised work-related mental injuries, ACC case managers contract occupational therapists (either through their local district health board or from the private sector) to work with the claimant's employer to develop a return-to-work plan. Claimants gain support in the time they have off work, with employers covering the worker's pay during the statutory amount of days. Employers are kept engaged during the entire vocational rehabilitation process. A gradual return to work is also possible.

The primary aim of the ACC process is to return eligible claimants to their preinjury job. This is not always possible, not the least because people may often lose their job during the rehabilitation process. In this case, various scenarios are possible. If the claimant's work capacity was restored successfully but the job was lost, ACC could offer a back-to-work programme and help the claimant find a new job. This would only cover a limited period, before a claimant would be referred to Work and Income. If a claimant develops an illness during the rehabilitation process which is not related to the initial accident, ACC cannot continue its support and entitlements and will transition the claimant to Work an Income.

For claimants who are unable to return to their pre-injury employment despite vocational rehabilitation, the aim of the ACC process is to achieve *vocational independence*, once an injury has healed or stabilised. The law in this case does not require restoring a claimant to an occupation of an economic and social status comparable to that before the injury or to take into account the actual current labour market realities (e.g. in cases where skills of a claimant are outdated). Once rendered vocationally independent, ACC payments are stopped after a period of another three months. Research has shown that just over half of those who were rendered vocationally independent actually returned to work (Armstrong and Laurs, 2007[41]) and that claimants' wage losses got larger the longer they have been out of work prior to being assessed as vocationally independent (Crichton, Stillman and Hyslop, 2005[42]).

De facto, however, vocational services are the exception: of all mental injury claims, for example, in 2016 only about 2.5% have gone through an initial occupational assessment and some 2% have received vocational rehabilitation services. This is also explained by the fact that far below 10% of all mental injury claims come from former workers; all other claims are from formerly inactive people. The share of claimants receiving vocational services is thus higher among other injury claims.

Expanding ACC to cover illness as well

Current ACC rules imply that effectively every year about 40 New Zealanders may receive vocational services in response to a mental injury claim, i.e. de facto no one. The potentially thousands of workers struggling with chronic often stress-related mental health conditions are excluded by definition and may often drop out of the labour market without receiving any such support. The same is true for an equally large number of physical illnesses of a chronic nature for which it is not possible to establish any causation with work and for all congenital disorders. This situation is disappointing: ACC has considerable resources and potential but not for the thousands of people who have mental health conditions, or other health conditions.

There are three options for the New Zealand government to change this situation. The first and grandest option is to revert to the Woodhouse principles underlying the introduction of ACC and to develop a system covering injuries and illnesses on an equal footing. This is not a new idea. It was the original intention when ACC was introduced, initially for injuries only to test the viability of the scheme but with the aim to include, at a later stage, all diseases. Only occupational diseases were included in the new scheme in 1972, importing the occupational-disease provisions from the previous Workers Compensation Act from 1956. It was also the plan pursued by the government of the time in 1989, following several Commission and Committee Reports (partly headed by Sir Owen Woodhouse), which was scrapped by the incoming government in 1990 (Duncan, $2016_{[43]}$). And extending the provision of ACC is also the aim of a new initiative currently explored by Warren Forster through a research grant by the Law Foundation at the occasion of the 50-year anniversary of the Woodhouse Report.

Expansion of ACC to cover all illnesses would require a reorientation of the health system, re-drawing the boundaries between the health, the welfare and the ACC system, and rethinking some of the rules and regulations, including the funding model. Expanding ACC is potentially costly. The risk to the financial sustainability to the scheme and the increased burden an expansion would likely place on both levy and tax payers is the main reason why policy makers are shying away from implementing the Woodhouse principles. However, transition costs could partly be offset by ACC's large reserve or investment fund and in the longer term, considerable savings can be realised from eliminating the costly process of identifying eligible injuries.[16]

A second, less costly option for New Zealand is a partial expansion of ACC. One of the principles of a partial expansion could be a shift in focus to work-related health problems. New Zealand has a long history of neglecting chronic health effects of work. Various authors have addressed the question of how coverage could be broadened to include chronic work-related health problems. Duncan ($2016_{[43]}$), for example, has argued that this also requires a shift in health and safety standards from safe work to healthy work, as argued in an earlier section of this chapter, as well as the development of a new set of enforcement tools.

Expanding ACC coverage for chronic work-related health problems certainly means it would cover a significant number of potentially stress-related mental health problems. This is a general challenge for Workers Compensation schemes around the world, which often struggle with this question. Systems in some countries are very rigorous: in Switzerland, for example, mental health conditions can only be covered if the claimant can prove that the illness was to at least 70% caused by work which is virtually impossible; accordingly, such cases hardly exist in Workers Compensation claims (OECD, $2014_{[33]}$). On the contrary, countries which are more lenient are recently seeing a massive increase in mental illness-related Workers Compensation claims; in Australia, mental illness claims today account for about 12% of all claims and – because of the often long-term nature of these claims – even one-third of total costs of the system (OECD, 2015[44]). It is in the hands of the legislator to decide what coverage level a system should provide.

The idea of a partial expansion of ACC is not new. Oliphant (2016[45]) has argued that the Woodhouse principles – which point to a universal scheme – are not helpful in thinking about partial expansion of ACC and that some mid-level principles are needed. In his view, any expansion should build on the idea that a public system must cover all those cases of incapacity that cannot legitimately be left to the private sphere, thus transgressing the boundary between injury and illness; congenital disorders in his line of argument, for example, should be covered by ACC.

A third option for New Zealand is to learn from ACC without expanding the coverage of the system itself. ACC is well placed to help people with injuries back into work at their own pace and over a long time, if necessary; and it achieves a return to work by involving all actors, including employers and general practitioners, in the process. It also has a comprehensive set of vocational services at hand, which it can use flexibly. No other institution in New Zealand is doing this in the same way. As much as possible, this approach and process could be replicated for cases of illness, especially mental health conditions, including very early intervention but also ongoing support, case management, effective return-to-work plans, access to integrated medical and vocational rehabilitation, and collaboration between employers and treating doctors. Other institutions, especially Work and Income, could adopt all of this for their clients.

Conclusion

New Zealand belongs to the group of OECD countries in which the link between mental health and work and the key role of the workplace are well understood, owing to long-run awareness-raising initiatives and the intellectual closeness to the United Kingdom where research on the health benefits of work is most advanced. However, that knowledge is not sufficiently reflected in policies and legislation. Partly this is because policy in relation to employers and workplaces is generally non-interventionist, similar to the United States and different from many European countries, and employment regulations therefore rather moderate and often leniently enforced. In order to help workers who are facing mental health challenges and to help employers who are struggling with health issues of their workforce, better policy and stricter enforcement and implementation of existing regulations is sometimes needed.

Health and safety at work legislation is a good example. While the intentions of recent reforms are laudable, regulations are not binding enough, implementation is weak, obligations of employers vague, and guidelines and supports for employers insufficient. Sickness policy is another example in case. Employer obligations vis-à-vis sick workers are mild and ineffective, public policy is largely inexistent compared to other countries, and the extent to which sick workers will receive support is therefore highly variable. Finally, regulations on work-related health problems are also problematic, putting people facing chronic stress and mental challenges at a particular disadvantage. This is a consequence of ACC reform in the 1970s, which cut a big divide between injury and illness and resulted in relatively poor care and support for everyone not eligible for ACC compensation and services (and, correspondingly, quite generous and effective support for those eligible for ACC).

People with mental health conditions are amongst those disadvantaged most from the structural weaknesses in the New Zealand system. Much could be done to improve the situation. Moving forward, special focus should be given to four aspects:

- How to expand the strengths of ACC to a larger part of the population;
- How to better support employers, especially small and medium-sized businesses;
- How to best support workers on sick leave with chronic (mental) health problems;
- How to strengthen the monitoring and implementation of existing legislation to improve outcomes and identify needs for further reform.

All of this will also require significantly improved data collection in a number of fields, especially including information on sickness absence, to make the Integrated Data Infrastructure more meaningful and useful to support the labour force participation of people with mental health conditions.

Notes

[1] Other data sources suggest that the prevalence of workplace bullying might be even higher. In a 2013 survey of the Public Service Association, one in three reported experiences of workplace bullying in the past six months. In a survey of employees across health, education, hospitality and travel sectors, the corresponding share was 18%. In a survey of the senior medical workforce, in 2017, 37% self-reported being bullied and two-thirds reported witnessing bullying of colleagues.

[2] The next national worker exposure survey, which was commissioned to Massey University, will include psychosocial questions to help address the absence of exposure data on psychosocial risk factors in New Zealand. Results are expected in February 2019.

[3] A serious work-related injury is one that results in hospitalisation and represents a probability of death (at admission) of at least 6.9%.

[4] WorkSafe is the prime health and safety regulator covering all workplaces in New Zealand apart from a few niche exceptions, which include work that takes place on seafaring vessels and in or around aircrafts and non-civilian workplaces operating under separate laws.

[5] https://worksafe.govt.nz/the-toolshed/tools/bullying-prevention-toolbox/

[6] In this context, the Canterbury Safety Charter is worth mentioning which was established with the help of WorkSafe. The charter is an agreement on health and safety between more than 370 organisations to ensure everyone involved in the post-quake rebuild goes home safe and healthy.

[7] The Mental Health Foundation also organises two national-level anti-stigma events each year with inputs into workplace mental health: *Mental Health Awareness Week* and *Pink Shirt Day*. The former runs over a week-long period in October, seeking to promote wellbeing in the workplace through a series of activities designed to disseminate information and stimulate discussion. The latter is a smaller-scale event focusing on promoting ideas around reducing workplace bullying and, more generally, promoting diversity. The Mental Health Foundation is also involved in a number of smaller-scale campaigns and events specific to certain regions or economic sectors.

[8] One initiative worth mentioning was Mindful Employer NZ, a pilot programme launched in one region of New Zealand in 2012, run by Platform Trust and Workwise and inspired by a similar programme in the United Kingdom (http://www.mindfulemployer.net/about/). The pilot, which was discontinued before it was scaled up, was dedicated to supporting employers and raising

awareness and understanding of mental health issues in the workplace, with a single point of information and navigation to resources on mental health.

[9] According to statistics for February 2016, 47% of the New Zealand workforce was employed in companies with more than 100 employees; 10% in those with 50-99 employees; 25% in those with 10-49 employees; 7% in those with 6-9 employees and 11% in those with 1-5 employees.

[10] The survey findings are based on a relatively small sample of 109 private and public business entities, which, however, well reflects the structure of the New Zealand workforce in terms of establishment size and industry structure. In total, the businesses in the sample employed 93 125 workers, of which 83 994 were permanent staff.

[11] While the government has no immediate plans to change the current provisions relating to sick leave, it has recently established a taskforce to review the Holidays Act and recommend changes to government. The scope is for a full review of the Act, focusing particularly on the provisions of, and payment for, holidays and leave entitlements, but with a remit to consider any other issues that arise in the course of the work of the taskforce.

[12] Regulations in New Zealand are very different in case of injuries. If an employee has an accident or injury covered by the ACC scheme, the following applies: a) If an employee has a work-related accident, the employer has to pay "first week compensation" equivalent to 80% of the employees' earnings; b) If an employee has a work-related or non-work-related accident and receives compensation from ACC, the employer cannot make the employee take time off as sick leave or annual holidays; c) If an employee is getting weekly compensation from ACC, the employer does not have to pay the employee; d) If the period of leave on ACC is more than five days, the employer and employee can agree that the employer will top up the ACC payment from 80% to 100% by using one day of employee's sick leave for every five days' leave taken.

[13] Note that the introduction of ACC cover for work-related mental injury, in 2008, came about partly in light of public outrage at the highly publicised case of Bruce Gardiner. He worked as a milk tanker driver in Hamilton and developed a post-traumatic stress disorder (and eventually went into medical retirement) following a work-related road accident in 2002 when a young man died after driving his car into the front of the milk tanker.

[14] While there are no plans currently to change ACCs approach towards coverage for mental health related injuries, the government is currently undertaking an analysis on the possibility of expanding mental injury cover for volunteer workers.

[15] It should be noted that the large majority of all ACC claims are short-term: only about 0.4% of all claimants were in receipt of weekly compensation for a period of six months or more.

[16] The no-blame feature of ACC has barred all suits for compensation for personal injury from the courts. However, instead ACC has created a large legal market of its own right engaged in distinguishing illness from injury and identifying eligible accidents. The total number of successful claims – almost two million claims for a population of less than five million – is telling: the incentive to lodge an ACC claim is tremendous and lawyers are often successful when they challenge a rejected claim.

References

ACC (2018), *Mental Injury Assessments for ACC*, ACC, Wellington, https://www.acc.co.nz/assets/provider/mental-injury-assessment-guide.pdf (accessed on 13 March 2018). [40]

Armstrong, H. and R. Laurs (2007), *Vocational Independence: outcomes for ACC claimants*, Department of Labour, Wellington, http://hazelarmstronglaw.co.nz/wp-content/uploads/2011/01/Vocational_Independence.pdf (accessed on 18 May 2018). [41]

Black, D. and D. Frost (2011), *Health at work – an independent review of sickness absence Dame Carol Black and David Frost CBE*, Department for Work and Pensions, London, https://assets.publishing.service.gov.uk/government/uploads/system/uploads/attachment_data/file/181060/health-at-work.pdf (accessed on 29 May 2018). [35]

BusinessNZ and Southern Cross Health Society (2017), *Wellness in the Workplace 2017: Survey Report*, Business New Zealand, Wellington, https://www.businessnz.org.nz/__data/assets/pdf_file/0009/128547/Wellness-in-the-Workplace-Survey-2017.pdf (accessed on 10 April 2018). [2]

Calder, K. et al. (2016), "Evaluation of a well-being campaign following a natural disaster in Christchurch, New Zealand", *International Journal of Mental Health Promotion*, Vol. 18/4, pp. 222-233, http://dx.doi.org/10.1080/14623730.2016.1210531. [16]

Crichton, S., S. Stillman and D. Hyslop (2005), *Returning to Work from Injury: Longitudinal Evidence on Employment and Earnings*, IZA Bonn, Bonn, http://repec.iza.org/dp1857.pdf (accessed on 18 May 2018). [42]

Department for Work and Pensions (2015), *Evaluation of the 2010–13 Fit for Work Service pilots: final report*, Department for Work and Pensions, https://assets.publishing.service.gov.uk/government/uploads/system/uploads/attachment_data/file/438234/rr896-fit-for-work-service-pilots.pdf (accessed on 18 May 2018). [39]

Drago, R. and K. Miller (2010), *Sick at Work: Infected Employees in the Workplace During the H1N1 Pandemic*, Institute for Women's Policy Research, Washington DC, https://iwpr.org/wp-content/uploads/wpallimport/files/iwpr-export/publications/B284.pdf (accessed on 29 May 2018). [22]

Duncan, D. (2016), "Regulating work that kills us slowly: The challenge of chronic work-related health problems", *New Zealand journal of employment relations.*, Vol. 41/2, pp. 87-103, https://search.informit.com.au/documentSummary;dn=372769667217146;res=IELNZC (accessed on 18 May 2018). [43]

Fergusson, D. et al. (2014), "Impact of a Major Disaster on the Mental Health of a Well-Studied Cohort", *JAMA Psychiatry*, Vol. 71/9, p. 1025, http://dx.doi.org/10.1001/jamapsychiatry.2014.652. [15]

Financial Services Council (2017), *Annual Report 2017*, Financial Services Council, https://www.fsc.org.nz/site/fsc/files/Statistics/2016/FSC%20Trad%20Risk%20Summary%202016-12.pdf (accessed on 18 May 2018). [28]

Gardner, D. et al. (2013), "Ethnicity, workplace bullying, social support and psychological strain in Aotearoa/New Zealand", *New Zealand Journal of Psychology*, Vol. 42/2, pp. 123-130, https://mro.massey.ac.nz/bitstream/handle/10179/9483/Gardner1%202013.pdf?sequence=1&isAllowed=y (accessed on 29 May 2018). [5]

Hargrave, G. et al. (2008), "EAP Treatment Impact on Presenteeism and Absenteeism: Implications for Return on Investment", *Journal of Workplace Behavioral Health*, Vol. 23/3, pp. 283-293, http://dx.doi.org/10.1080/15555240802242999. [30]

Health Promotion Agency (2018), *Wellbeing and Mental Distress in Aotearoa New Zealand: Snapshot 2016*, Health Promotion Agency, Wellington, https://www.hpa.org.nz/sites/default/files/Wellbeing-And-Mental-Distress-Snapshot-2016-Final-FEB2018.PDF (accessed on 10 April 2018). [3]

Independent Taskforce on Workplace Health and Safety (2013), *The report of Independent Taskforce on Workplace Health and Safety*, Independent Taskforce on Workplace Health and Safety, Wellington, http://hstaskforce.govt.nz/documents/report-of-the-independent-taskforce-on-workplace-health-safety.pdf (accessed on 09 April 2018). [7]

Independent Taskforce on Workplace Health and Safety (2013), *WORKPLACE HEALTH & SAFETY*, http://hstaskforce.govt.nz/documents/report-of-the-independent-taskforce-on-workplace-health-safety.pdf (accessed on 03 October 2018). [8]

Kausto, J. et al. (2014), "Effectiveness of new legislation on partial sickness benefit on work participation: a quasi-experiment in Finland.", *BMJ open*, Vol. 4/12, p. e006685, http://dx.doi.org/10.1136/bmjopen-2014-006685. [36]

Kendall, N. et al. (2015), *Developing an intervention toolbox for common health problems in the workplace*, Health and Safety Executive, London, http://www.hse.gov.uk/research/rrpdf/rr1053.pdf (accessed on 29 May 2018). [27]

Lam, R. and A. Walker (2012), "The Prevalence and Impact of Depression in Self-Referred Clients Attending an Employee Assistance Program", *Journal of Occupational and Environmental Medicine*, Vol. 54/11, pp. 1395-1399, http://dx.doi.org/10.1097/JOM.0b013e3182611a69. [31]

Martin, D. (2015), *Worksafe New Zealand: Targeted Independent Review*, Ministry of Business, Innovation and Employment, http://www.mbie.govt.nz/info-services/employment-skills/workplace-health-and-safety-reform/document-and-image-library/Targeted%20independent%20review.pdf (accessed on 10 April 2018). [13]

MBIE (2013), *Working Safer: A blueprint for health and safety at work*, New Zealand Government, Wellington, http://www.mbie.govt.nz/info-services/employment-skills/workplace-health-and-safety-reform/document-and-image-library/working-safer-key-documents/safety-first-blueprint.pdf (accessed on 14 March 2018). [6]

Mental Health Foundation (2017), *Let's Make Mental Health Part of the Conversation: A Guide for Managers*, Mental Health Foundation of New Zealand, Auckland, https://www.mentalhealth.org.nz/assets/Uploads/Guide-for-managers-April-2017.pdf (accessed on 23 March 2018). [18]

Mental Health Foundation (2016), *Working Well: A workplace guide to mental health*, Mental Health Foundation of New Zealand, Auckland, https://www.mentalhealth.org.nz/assets/Our-Work/Open-Minds/Working-Well-guide.pdf (accessed on 23 March 2018). [20]

Mental Health Foundation and Health Promotion Agency (2018), *Five Ways to Wellbeing at Work: Toolkit*, Mental Health Foundation of New Zealand, Auckland, https://www.mentalhealth.org.nz/assets/Uploads/Five-Ways-to-Wellbeing-at-Worknew2018.pdf (accessed on 23 March 2018). [19]

Milli, J., J. Xia and J. Min (2016), *Paid Sick Days Benefit Employers, Workers, and the Economy Employers Benefit from Paid Sick Days*, Institute for Women's Policy Research, Washington DC, https://iwpr.org/wp-content/uploads/wpallimport/files/iwpr-export/publications/B361.pdf (accessed on 29 May 2018). [23]

OECD (2015), *Fit Mind, Fit Job: From Evidence to Practice in Mental Health and Work*, OECD Publishing, Paris, http://dx.doi.org/10.1787/9789264228283-en. [1]

OECD (2015), *Mental Health and Work: Australia*, Mental Health and Work, OECD Publishing, Paris, http://dx.doi.org/10.1787/9789264246591-en. [44]

OECD (2015), *Mental Health and Work: Austria*, Mental Health and Work, OECD Publishing, Paris, http://dx.doi.org/10.1787/9789264228047-en. [47]

OECD (2015), *Recommendation of the Council on Integrated Mental Health, Skills and Work Policy*, OECD Publications, Paris, https://legalinstruments.oecd.org/Instruments/ShowInstrumentView.aspx?InstrumentID=334&Lang=en&Book=False (accessed on 08 February 2018). [4]

OECD (2014), *Mental Health and Work: Netherlands*, Mental Health and Work, OECD Publishing, Paris, http://dx.doi.org/10.1787/9789264223301-en. [34]

OECD (2014), *Mental Health and Work: Switzerland*, Mental Health and Work, OECD Publishing, Paris, http://dx.doi.org/10.1787/9789264204973-en. [33]

OECD (2014), *Mental Health and Work: United Kingdom*, Mental Health and Work, OECD Publishing, Paris, http://dx.doi.org/10.1787/9789264204997-en. [38]

OECD (2013), *Mental Health and Work: Belgium*, Mental Health and Work, OECD Publishing, Paris, http://dx.doi.org/10.1787/9789264187566-en. [10]

OECD (2013), *Mental Health and Work: Denmark*, Mental Health and Work, OECD Publishing, Paris, http://dx.doi.org/10.1787/9789264188631-en. [14]

OECD (2013), *Mental Health and Work: Norway*, Mental Health and Work, OECD Publishing, Paris, http://dx.doi.org/10.1787/9789264178984-en. [32]

OECD (2013), *Mental Health and Work: Sweden*, Mental Health and Work, OECD Publishing, Paris, http://dx.doi.org/10.1787/9789264188730-en. [37]

OECD (2013), *OECD Employment Outlook 2013*, OECD Publishing, Paris, http://dx.doi.org/10.1787/empl_outlook-2013-en. [29]

Oliphant, K. (2016), "BEYOND WOODHOUSE: DEVISING NEW PRINCIPLES FOR DETERMINING ACC BOUNDARY ISSUES", *Victoria University of Wellington Law Review*, Vol. 35/4, pp. 915-936, http://orca.cf.ac.uk/66841/1/oliphant.pdf (accessed on 18 May 2018). [45]

Raub, A. et al. (2018), *Paid Leave for Personal Illness: A Detailed Look at Approaches Across OECD Countries*, WORLD Policy Analysis Center, Los Angeles, https://www.worldpolicycenter.org/sites/default/files/WORLD%20Report%20-%20Personal%20Medical%20Leave%20OECD%20Country%20Approaches_0.pdf (accessed on 29 May 2018). [26]

Social Security Administration (2016), *Social Security Programs Throughout the World: Europe, 2016*, Social Security Administration, https://www.ssa.gov/policy/docs/progdesc/ssptw/2016-2017/europe/ssptw16europe.pdf (accessed on 18 May 2018). [25]

Spasova, S., D. Bouget and B. Vanhercke (2016), *Sick pay and sickness benefit schemes in the European Union Background report for the Social Protection Committee's*, European Commission, Brussels, http://KE-02-17-045-EN-N (1).pdf. [24]

State Services Commission (2016), *Worker Wellness Information and Resources*, Government of New Zealand, Wellington, https://www.ssc.govt.nz/sites/all/files/worker-wellness-resource-kit_0.pdf (accessed on 10 April 2018). [46]

Thornicroft, G. et al. (2016), "Evidence for effective interventions to reduce mental-health-related stigma and discrimination.", *The Lancet (London, England)*, Vol. 387/10023, pp. 1123-1132, http://dx.doi.org/10.1016/S0140-6736(15)00298-6. [17]

Vester Thorsen, S. et al. (2015), *Sickness absence in the Nordic Countries*, Nordic Social Statistical Committee, Copenhagen, http://norden.diva-portal.org/smash/get/diva2:811504/FULLTEXT06.pdf (accessed on 04 April 2018). [21]

WorkSafe (2016), *Healthy Work: Work-related health strategic plan*, WorkSafe, Wellington, https://worksafe.govt.nz/topic-and-industry/work-related-health/work-related-health-strategic-plan/ (accessed on 14 March 2018). [11]

WorkSafe (2016), *Introduction to the Health and Safety at Work Act: Special guide*, New Zealand Government, Wellington, https://worksafe.govt.nz/managing-health-and-safety/getting-started/introduction-hswa-special-guide/ (accessed on 12 March 2018). [9]

WorkSafe and ACC (2016), *Safer. Healthier. Together: An Action Plan 2016-2019 - Reducing Harm in New Zealand Workplaces*, New Zealand Government, Wellington, https://www.acc.co.nz/assets/business/action-plan-reduce-harm-NZ-workplaces.pdf (accessed on 14 March 2018) [12]

Chapter 5. Social protection measures and employment services in New Zealand

This chapter evaluates policies and programmes aimed at improving the responsiveness of New Zealand's social protection system and employment services to people with mental health conditions. It considers how this system ensures secure income in periods of inactivity, how it recognises and responds to people with mental health conditions and how the system helps people out of work to return to the labour market. The analysis uses the OECD's (2015) Council Recommendation on Integrated Mental Health, Skills and Work Policy *as the primary benchmark for informing best practice policies in this field.*

Introduction

Across OECD countries, mental health conditions account for the bulk of new and existing claims for health and disability benefits. These claims are different from most of the claims for people with physical complaints. The reason lies in the very nature of mental health conditions – onset at an earlier age, high recurrence, fluctuating course, as well as frequent comorbidities with other health issues. The consequence is a much greater labour market distance, with frequent periods of unemployment and inactivity. Compounding this is poor knowledge in the unemployment system of how to recognise and respond to mental health issues and frequently an underestimation of peoples' capacity to work. In OECD countries, this is reflected in limited benefit outflows and high disability claims because of incorrect allocation to the right intensity of employment assistance at the right time.

It is important to identify mental health symptoms and resulting labour market barriers as early as possible – ideally, on a jobseeker's first contact with the welfare system, or soon after. The longer a person is out of work the harder and costlier it is to support them to return to work. Periods out of work should be as short as possible. Where a mental health issue is identified or suspected, case management support should involve health expertise to facilitate swift access to appropriate health treatment, as necessary, in parallel with an effective return-to-work strategy.

Mental health competence and psychological expertise in the employment sector, however, are generally underdeveloped and not commensurate with the high prevalence of mental health conditions among jobseekers and welfare clients. These competencies have to be strengthened to make early identification and quick intervention possible in all systems. Efforts in that direction should come in the unemployment system especially because better job retention and reintegration at this early stage can prevent people with poor mental health from slipping into longer-term welfare dependence and disability.

The main challenges for the social protection and employment services system

The OECD *Recommendation of the Council on Integrated Mental Health, Skills and Work Policy* calls upon its member countries to: "seek to improve the responsiveness of social protection systems and employment services to the needs of people living with mental health conditions", detailing key priorities for action policy makers should consider. Table 2.1 gives an assessment of New Zealand's performance against the OECD Council Recommendations, and suggested actions. In summary:

The structural reforms to the welfare system have been unsuccessful in reducing the number of people with mental health conditions claiming health and disability benefits, and these claims continue to rise, particularly amongst Māori and Pacific people. Māori people are overrepresented in claims for all main benefits, making up 31% of all people on benefits, 25% of Supported Living Payment claimants for mental health reasons and 23% of Job Seekers Allowance claimants for mental health reasons. The numbers and rise of Māori people with mental health problems on benefit is a major concern and addressing this should be a priority. Welfare reforms have not helped in reducing ethnic inequities.

Table 5.1. New Zealand's performance regarding the OECD Council Recommendations around improving the social protection system's response to mental health conditions

	OECD Council Recommendation	New Zealand's performance	Suggested actions
A	Reduce preventable disability benefit claims for mental health conditions through **recognition of the work capacity of those potentially claiming a benefit**, and through a focus on early identification and early provision of medical and/or vocational support as necessary.	People with mental health conditions make up the majority of claims for health and disability benefits. Māori are overrepresented in health and disability benefits. Little focus on early intervention, with current assessment processes not necessarily picking up mental health issues.	Comprehensive allocation and navigation process for quicker and effective matching to right psychological and employment support. Assessment and case management need to be inclusive of Māori models of practice based on a practice philosophy of Whānau Ora. Employment services need to better support people whilst they are working. Evaluate the experience of people with mental health conditions in the employment system.
B	Help jobseekers living with mental health conditions into work through **appropriate outreach tools** as well as services that address the labour market barriers associated with a jobseeker's mental health condition.	The system underestimates the numbers of people with mental health conditions on benefits. Case management and support is not offered actively to all MSD clients or matched to their need. There is a lack of access to psychological support. The distinction between JS-WR, JS-HCD and SLP is unhelpful.	The benefits system needs simplifying. Evaluate the assessment processes to inform a new process with timely and appropriate follow up psychological and employment support offered to all MSD clients. Remove access restrictions for employment support services i.e. diagnosis, benefits status. Increase access to psychological therapies for people claiming benefits. Access to therapies should include Māori health practitioners.
C	Invest in **mental health competences for those administering the social protection system** by providing training for staff by ensuring co-operation of benefit and employment services with psychological services.	Mental health training is available to MSD staff. There is too little involvement of allied health professionals. There is little communication from Work & Income back to primary care practitioners.	Make mental health competency training mandatory for all MSD staff and integrate cultural responses to mental health within this, including Māori models of practice. Expand training, focus on the interrelationship between mental health and work. MSD staff needs earlier and greater access to health advisors with mental health expertise.
D	Encourage the **integration of mental health treatment into employment service delivery** by stimulating cooperation with the health sector and the development of evidence-based vocational interventions for jobseekers with common mental health conditions	Promising pilots but these have been going for six years. Funding of employment services for people with mental health conditions is fragmented, insufficient and short term. Move to outcomes payments is a positive step, but contract design needs to reward the provision of evidence-based practices. Individual Placement & Support (IPS) services are available only in some regions.	Implement a national mental health and employment strategy. Coordinate service procurement between MOH and MSD, and within MSD. Scale up vocational interventions that integrate psychological support and incorporate Māori models of practice. Increase the availability of IPS services. Monitor adherence to the national guidelines for employment support providers. Extend contract duration and provide financial incentives for evidence-based practices and the provision of post-placement support.

Source: Authors' own assessment based on all of the evidence collected in this chapter.

Better assessment and support systems are needed which quickly identify mental health issues across all people claiming benefits regardless of primary reason for claim, and support people to access integrated psychological and employment support services. The pathway to early and appropriate employment assistance and psychological support is unclear, inconsistent and inequitable.

Employment support services need expanding to people with mental health issues who are not claiming benefits to prevent hardship and higher societal costs later on.

The mental health competencies of staff working in the welfare system need further strengthening, building on the already available mental health training. Training should be mandatory, comprehensive and culturally informed. Case managers also need to increase their understanding of psychological techniques and have quick and easy access to psychological coaching and support services.

The employment sector needs strengthening. The non-government employment sector is underfunded, characterised by short-term pilots and as a result service provision is fragmented and access inequitable. Within the public employment service there is a significant mismatch between individual employment assistance needs and the intensity of case management support people actually receive.

A national mental health and employment strategy that addresses policy and funding barriers and helps to build national coverage of evidence-based employment services integrated with mental health treatment should be developed and implemented.

Overview of New Zealand's social protection system

New Zealand established the Welfare State with the enactment of the Social Security Act in 1938. Social welfare is mostly funded through general taxation and, since the 1980s, income support has been provided based on need, except for universal superannuation (state pension for people from the age of 65).

Work and Income New Zealand (Work and Income) provides employment services and income support throughout the country on behalf of the Ministry of Social Development. Work and Income administers the payment of social benefits, supports jobseekers into employment and contracts with non-government employment-service providers (see Box 5.1 for more details on the New Zealand social protection system).

In 2012, under the previous government and led by the Treasury and the State Services Commission, *Better Public Services* a cross-government initiative was introduced (Public Services Advisory Group, 2011[1]). *Better Public Services* consisted of ten high-level targets with specific results-oriented goals for the government to attain over time. Relevant targets contained within the strategy were around reducing long-term welfare dependence (Result 1) and setting strong foundations for work and life – primarily focusing on skills development (Results 5 and 6).

As part of the drive to reduce future welfare liability, from 2010, the former government set in place a series of welfare reforms including in 2013 specific health and disability reforms, recognising that most people can and do want to work (Work and Income, 2013[2]). The reforms included a change to obligations and to the income support benefits. In 2010, obligations were introduced to some people on Sickness Benefit. In 2013, Sickness Benefit was brought into a new benefit, Jobseekers Support, which is for all jobseekers, and contains sub-categories: Jobseekers with a Health Condition or Disability (JS-HCD), and Jobseekers who are Work Ready (JS-WR). At the same time, Invalid's Benefit was replaced with the Supported Living Payment (SLP). People claiming Invalid's Benefit had no obligations attached, but after the welfare reforms, some people on SLP now also have work-preparation obligations (see Box 5.2 for more details on the 2013 Health and Disability Welfare Reforms).

Box 5.1. About the New Zealand social protection system

The initial point of contact for anyone who is seeking financial assistance and employment services is through Work & Income New Zealand (Work and Income), Te Hiranga Tangata. Work and Income is a public one-stop shop and a business unit within the Ministry of Social Development, Te Manatū Whakahiato Ora. Work and Income services include skills development, work-search support, income support and in-work support, and helping people to secure childcare. Work and Income is divided into 11 regions, with 160 service centres across the country, serving around 294 000 each week, and paying out more than NZD 8 billion annually in financial support. Work and Income employs around 2 500 staff.

The New Zealand social protection and employment service system is predominantly provided by government, through Work and Income, with around 17% of the operational budget contracted to non-government providers. As part of the recent welfare reforms, Work and Income adopted a case management approach to provide a range of general and work-focused services according to client need. The primary role of case management is to reduce long-term welfare dependence by increasing labour market participation. In 2014 there were 1 780 full-time equivalent case managers.

Over recent years, the welfare system has adopted an investment approach aligned with that used in the insurance industry. The investment approach predicts the likely long-term benefits costs of a person based on what has happened in the past to other people with similar background and circumstances. It works out what interventions and services work best and for whom, and it uses this information to set priorities for investment (and disinvestment) and direct services to those people most likely to achieve positive change. The current government is reconsidering this approach.

There are three main benefits for people out of work: Jobseeker Support, Supported Living Payment and Sole Parent Support. The rates of payment vary according to individuals' marital status, age and number of dependents (Table 5.2). Eligibility for income support depends on partner's employment status, other income sources and assets.

Table 5.2. Benefits rates and obligations, for single adults, no children, as at April 2018

Benefit type	Net weekly rate after tax	Obligations
Jobseekers support (work-ready)	NZD 215.34[a]	Full-time work obligations: To find or prepare for work of at least 30 hours per week, take part in work-ability assessments, interviews, meetings and assessments if the person has been referred to a Contracted service provider
Jobseeker support (HC-D)	NZD 215.34[a]	Part-time work obligations: To find or prepare for work of at least 15 hours per week. Some people claiming JS (HC-D) will be exempt from work obligations and may only have work preparation obligations.
Supported Living Payment	NZD 269.15[b]	Work preparation obligations: To attend - interviews to determine capacity to engage in work preparation; work ability assessments; participate in interviews and activities with Contracted Service Providers when this has been agreed.
Sole Parent Support	NZD 334.05	Part-time work obligations when your youngest child is aged 3-13 (unless you have a health condition or disability); Work preparation obligations when your youngest child is under 3. Take part in work ability assessments and activities with Contracted Service Providers.

a) Single 25 years or older no children, b) Single 18 years or older, without children.
Source: (MSD, 2018[3]).

Box 5.2. The 2013 Health and Disability Welfare Reforms

In seeking to reduce future welfare liabilities, the Government focused the most recent reforms on people not participating in the labour market. This was because between June 2004 and June 2014, the number of people not available for work had increased by nearly 64 100 to just more than 1.1 million, almost one-third of the working-age population.

There were three stages to the 2011 to 2013 reforms. In 2012, support for young people changed to encourage young people back into education or training. The second reforms focused on sole parents, widows and other women alone. In 2013, the biggest changes took place. The 2013 Health and Disability Welfare Reforms collapsed all previous main benefits into three categories, extended work-focused interventions to a wider range of people and introduced additional obligations for some people to meet.

There are two main benefit types for people with identified health conditions and disabilities, including people with mental health conditions: **Jobseeker Support on the grounds of health condition or disability** (JS-HCD) and **Supported Living Payment** (SLP). Access to these benefits is granted on the basis of the impact the health condition or disability has on the person's ability to work, not the existence of the health condition or disability itself. SLP is a slightly higher weekly benefit than JS-HCD. For example for a single adult 25 years or older, they would receive a payment of NZD 265.54 per week on SLP, and NZD 212.45 per week on JS-HCD. There is no difference in payment for a person claiming JS-HCD and a person claiming JS (work ready).

To receive **Jobseeker Support** on the ground of a health condition, injury or disability, a person must be limited in their capacity or unable to work full-time due to a health condition, injury or disability; or in employment but because of a health condition, injury or disability unable to work or only at a reduced level.

JS-HCD is a temporary benefit, with the impact of a health condition on work capacity expected to last less than two years. People whose capacity to work is permanently but only partially restricted to having a capacity for between 15 and 29 hours of work per week can also receive JS.

People in receipt of JS-HCD may have their work obligations deferred. When a client is applying for (or transfers to) JC-HCD they need to provide a current medical certificate, based on a medical review. The first certificate covers up to a maximum of four weeks. After the first four weeks, a second review is needed, again covering up to a maximum of four weeks. After eight weeks, a third review is required covering a maximum of 13 weeks. A medical certificate is required thereafter every 13 weeks, and a person must reapply for JS after 52 weeks, since this is a temporary, work-focused payment.

Abatement rates apply when a person reaches a certain level of income, including through earnings, resulting in reduced benefit payment (partial). People can work up to 30 hours per week (depending on abatement levels) before they are no longer considered eligible for JS.

Supported Living Payment (SLP) is for people not able to work because they are permanently and severely restricted in their capacity for work because of a health condition, injury, or disability, or fully blind. Permanent means the health condition, injury or disability a person has is expected to continue for at least two years, or the claimant has been diagnosed with a terminal illness. Severely means a client cannot regularly work 15 hours or more per week in open employment. Work preparation obligations are legislated but not used in practice for people receiving SLP. Abatement rates apply when a person reaches a certain level of income, including through earnings, resulting in reduced benefit payment.

Disability Allowance

The Disability Allowance provides non-taxable assistance to people who have on-going, additional costs because of a disability, including mental health. This assistance is available to people on benefit and non-beneficiaries with low income (provided they meet the income thresholds). The amount payable is based on the additional costs of disability up to a maximum amount per week.

Assessment process

The Health and Disability Welfare Reforms include a new staged assessment process for people with a health condition or a disability to identify their ability to work. This includes:

- Enabling people with very little or no work capacity, or whose condition is deteriorating or will not improve, or who are terminally ill, to receive benefit without any requirement for additional assessments of their ability to work.
- A self-assessment questionnaire to collect the person's view on their ability to work and the supports and services they need to prepare for, or find and stay in, work.
- A medical certification process with focus on what a person can do at work with appropriate services and supports. People are required to submit a medical certificate at four weeks, eight weeks and then every 13 weeks.
- An assessment of work ability (including on-going assessment through structured interviews during case management services), and, if earlier less intensive approaches (i.e. the self-assessment and structured interview) have not given clarity about what someone can do or the help they need to work, an independent Work Ability Assessment (WAA).

People may also be required to attend an appointment with a designated doctor as part of a second-opinion process. MSD does not track outcomes as such but from a qualitative view, it knows that there are opportunities to improve on this, which is part of the work under the Health and Disability work programme.

Source: Authors own compilation using OAG (2014[3]) and Productivity Commission (2015[4]).

The welfare reforms also saw Work and Income set in place a case management approach, employing three types of case managers: general, work-focused and work-search support case managers (Figure 5.1). General and work-focused case managers both check and process clients' benefit entitlements, make referrals to other social support and apply sanctions if clients do not meet their obligations. Work-focused and work-search support case managers also help clients to search a job, refer to training as required and work with clients to find solutions to issues preventing them from working. Work-search support case managers deliver seminars and provide other types of training to help job seekers. Case manager consistency allows building a relationship; this can be critical for the outcome.

Accordingly, work-focused case managers have multiple, potentially conflicting roles: supporting financial assistance, providing employment support, and imposing sanctions when clients do not meet their obligations. In other countries, the decision to impose sanctions comes from a higher level, to remove any conflicting roles for frontline workers. New Zealand could consider this.[1]

Clients are matched to case management services based on client information (such as the type of benefit, age, location, previous benefit history), analytics (predictive modelling) and agreed business rules (certain conditions may exclude a person from service) that prioritises clients to services based on eligibility and availability in each Work and Income service centre. This also includes a case management service for clients with health conditions or disabilities.

Figure 5.1. An illustration of Work and Income's case management approach

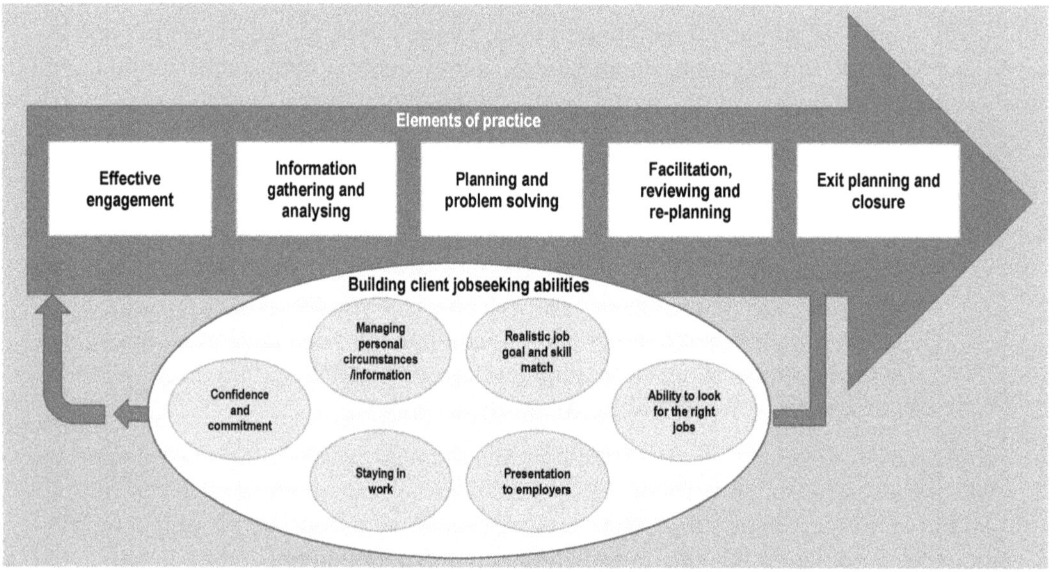

Source: Adapted from: OAG (2014), Ministry of Social Development: using a case management approach to service delivery, Wellington: Office of the Auditor General.

In May 2018, MSD launched a trial in four sites where clients are given the choice to opt in. Clients are provided with information about the services Work and Income can offer and can select the one they believe is right for them. Clients can discuss the alternative options with their case managers but the decision rests firmly with the client. The aim of the trial is for clients to feel more empowered and engaged and having greater choice is a core part of that. The trial will be evaluated through feedback from the service centres and the clients involved.

In 2014, an audit of the case management approach found that although overall the system was working well, MSD was not working in a co-ordinated way with other sectors to address the multiple needs of people with the highest barriers to employment (OAG, 2014[3]). This audit found that their needs to be a greater focus on supporting the development of case managers' soft skills, such as effective client engagement, alongside their technical skills, and the need to focus on compliance.

A follow up review three years later found that progress had been made to strengthen the capacity of case managers, including training in active listening, communication and empathy, however, accuracy in their processing skills still strongly influenced case managers' performance ratings. The report also found that MSD had not progressed the sector response required to better support working-age adults with higher or complex needs, even though it had progressed its own initiatives in this area (OAG, 2017[5]). Building the mental health and cultural competency of case managers, and increasing access to mental health practitioners, could go some way to address this recommendation.

Benefit claims due to mental health conditions are increasing

Since the welfare reforms, MSD has commissioned annual valuation reports on the benefits system. The 2016 evaluation had a specific section on people with mental health conditions. This identified that the average future lifetime liability of this client group is significantly higher than of the average client with a health condition or disability, NZD 33 000 higher for clients on JS-HCD and NZD 52 000 for clients on SLP (Greenfield, Miller and Mcguire, 2016[6]). The report argued that this difference was due mainly to the younger age of people who claim for mental health conditions compared to other clients claiming for health conditions and disabilities.

Whilst the reforms have reduced the overall numbers of people of working age claiming welfare benefits (Greenfield, Miller and Mcguire, 2016[6]), the numbers of people claiming benefits whose primary reason for claiming is a mental health condition, has continued to rise. Of SLP claimants, in December 2012 mental health claims made up 31% of claims, and by December 2017 this had risen to 35% (a rise from 25 883 to 29 567 people). Similarly, claims for mental health conditions within people claiming JS-HCD grew from 42.5% in December 2012 to 47.9% in December 2017 (an increase from 26 026 to 27 512 people), (Figure 5.2) (MSD, 2018[7]; MSD, 2017[8]).

The increase in the proportion of people claiming due to mental health conditions is in part related to the fact that the overall numbers of claimants on JS-HCD has reduced (from 61 245 in 2012 to 57 428 in 2017). The increase in numbers may in part be due to an increasing prevalence of mental health conditions in the population (Potter et al., 2017). However, more likely it is an indication that the reforms have not been as successful in supporting clients with mental health conditions – who face multiple barriers to employment – off benefit and into work, especially when compared to people with other health conditions or disabilities. Data shows that with the exception of cancer and congenital conditions, claims for mental health reasons is the only health and disability client group to have increased in numbers in the past five years (MSD, 2017[8]).

Figure 5.2. Welfare benefits claims for mental health reasons continue to increase

Share of MSD clients with a mental health condition as the primary reason for claiming

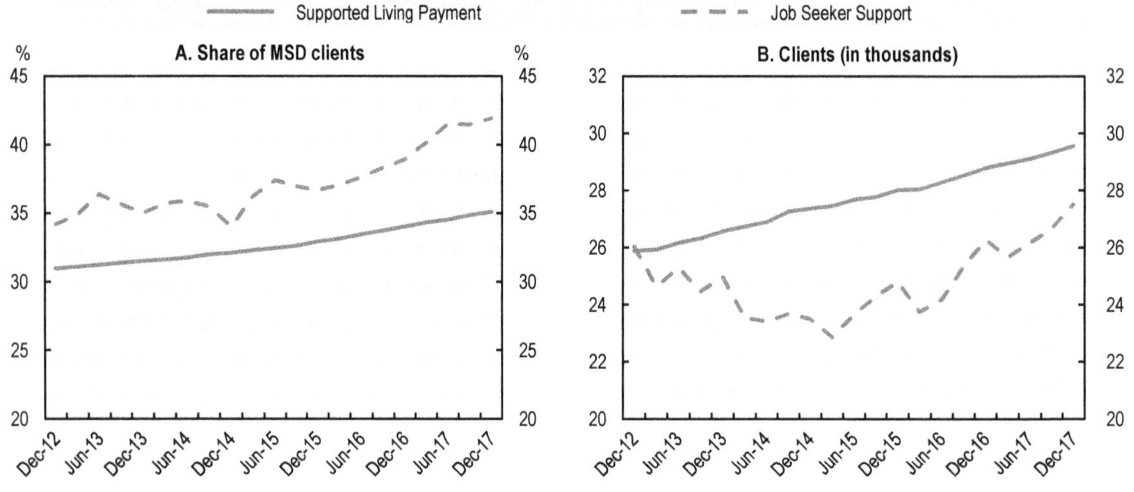

Source: Ministry of Social Development (2017) *Quarterly benefits Tables December 2017.*

StatLink http://dx.doi.org/10.1787/888933845643

Figure 5.2 (Panel B) further shows that there are as many people claiming JS-HCD for mental health reasons as are people claiming SLP for mental health reasons, with some systematic differences in the composition of the two groups.

Claims due to mental health conditions cover a range of issues. Claims coded as stress and depression make up a significant proportion, 41%, of mental health claims for JS-HCD. People diagnosed with bipolar disorder and schizophrenia represent a larger proportion of claims for mental health reasons for SLP, at 47% (Greenfield, Miller and Mcguire, 2016[6]).

People claiming benefits for mental health reasons are also younger than the average person claiming a government payment. For instance, the average age of people claiming JS-HCD for mental health reasons is 7.6 years younger than for other JS-HCD clients; the corresponding figure is 4.4 years for SLP clients. Claims for mental health conditions are uneven across age groups. For example, as at October 2017, mental health claims made up 48% of claims for SLP for people aged under 25 and 70% for clients under 25 claiming JS-HCD (Greenfield, Miller and Mcguire, 2016[6]).

Ethnic inequities among mental health related claims are large and growing

Māori people are overrepresented in claims for all benefits. They comprise 31% of all benefits claims, but only 15% of the working-age population. In 2016, Māori people made up 25% of people claiming SLP for mental health reasons and 23% of people claiming JS-HCD for mental health reasons. They also stay on benefits longer regardless of the type of benefit and service they receive (MSD, 2018[7]). The numbers of Māori people claiming JS-HCD and SLP for mental health reasons is also increasing (Figure 5.3, Panel A).

Pacific people make up 5% of all people on SLP; 7% of those on JS-HCD; 4% of people claiming SLP for mental health reasons and 3% of people claiming JS-HCD for mental health reasons. This compares with a share in the total working-age population, in 2017, corresponding to 7%. The numbers of Pacific people claiming benefits for mental health reasons is also increasing (Figure 5.3, Panel B).

Figure 5.3. Gradual increase in the number of Māori and Pacific people claiming benefits for mental health reasons

Current recipients of JS-HCD and SLP for mental health reasons

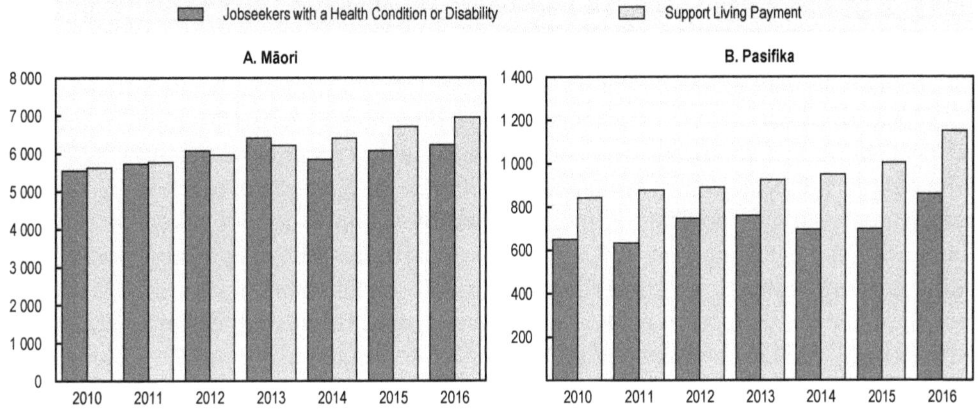

Source: Administrative data supplied by the Ministry of Social Development.

StatLink http://dx.doi.org/10.1787/888933845662

Analysis of mental health claims by ethnicity further highlights the ethnic disparities, with the rates of increase over time much higher for Māori and Pacific people compared with New Zealand European (Table 5.3).

Table 5.3. Trends in mental health claim numbers vary remarkably by ethnicity

	2010	2016	Difference	Rate of change
JS-HCD mental health condition				
Māori	5 550	6 223	673	12%
Pacific	650	859	209	32%
NZ European	14 020	12 724	-1 296	-9%
Other	3 046	3 754	708	23%
Unspecified	665	632	-33	-5%
Total	**23 931**	**24 192**	**261**	**1%**
SLP mental health condition				
Māori	5 630	6 953	1 323	24%
Pacific	842	1 150	308	37%
NZ European	14 793	15 290	497	3%
Other	3 325	3 781	456	14%
Unspecified	378	335	-43	-11%
Total	**24 968**	**27 509**	**2 541**	**10%**

Source: Administrative data supplied by the Ministry of Social Development.

StatLink http://dx.doi.org/10.1787/888933845719

Changes over time indicate that whilst there is some reduction in numbers of NZ Europeans claiming JS-HCD for mental health reasons, the numbers of Māori and Pacific people claiming benefits for mental health reasons is continuing to rise.

A large share of clients have been on health and disability benefits over two years

A large proportion of people are also claiming benefits for more than two years: some 44% of people claiming JS-HCD and nearly all people claiming SLP. This data further highlights the importance of acting quickly to provide access to mental health treatment and employment assistance when people are not yet disconnected from the labour market (and thus receiving JS-WR) and the importance of supporting people into employment even earlier, prior to becoming MSD clients.

MSD clients with mental health conditions might desire to work but hesitate to seek it if it might jeopardise their current entitlements. Anecdotal evidence from people in receipt of benefits suggests that some see the system as opaque and do not understand whether they will be able to get back onto a benefit easily if they take a chance to look for work and therefore many of the poorest or most vulnerable simply do not take the risk. This concurs with the findings from an MSD survey of over 400 people and organisations working across the health and disability sector who commented when asked what could reduce the financial disincentives to working was "make the system easier to understand" (MSD, 2014[9]). MSD is currently in the process of trying to ensure people understand the benefit system, and that they receive the payment they are, in principle, eligible for.

The benefits system itself therefore appears to create certain tangible disincentives for work. This is particularly problematic when people want to work and can with the right support. For example, JS-HCD incentivises fulltime work (30 hours or more) and therefore does not encourage a graduated return to work. SLP abates at a rate of 70 cents to the dollar after a beneficiary has earnt up to NZD 200 per week and this creates a disincentive to work more than 15 hours a week. Claimants with fluctuating conditions and support needs are likely to be fearful of moving off SLP in case employment does not work out. The current SLP Sustainable Employment Trial only allows people to try working 15 hours or more a week for 26 weeks (this period may be increased to two years in future trials). MSD is currently examining how to make changes to the benefit system to include smooth transitions in and out of benefits, and to improve awareness and take up of some of the existing incentives that are already available. Any changes need to consider the relevant differences between SLP and JS-HCD; and how these differences may create additional barriers, or encourage certain behaviours, among people working in the system, as well as those accessing it.

Organisations providing support services for people with disabilities, including people with mental health conditions, argue that what is needed is an employment strategy instead of the predominant benefit-reduction strategy (NZDSN, 2016[10]; NZDSN, 2015[11]).[2] This is an important point, as realigning the strategy to a genuine employment strategy would introduce a new way of thinking and working across the system. A mental health and employment strategy could include how to set up and support relapse prevention plans, working well plans and whānau ora plans, once people are in employment. The current New Zealand Disability Strategy reinforces this need to focus on employment outcomes over benefits reduction, for people with disabilities. An employment strategy is one of the eight key outcomes of the strategic plan (ODI, 2016[12]).

Furthermore, the New Zealand system appears as a highly unequal system, with higher benefits (in terms of income replacement) and faster access to health, employment and training services for people falling under ACC (see Chapters 1, 2 and 4 for more information on ACC). In contrast, people being out of work for health-related issues have to manage on savings and, once depleted, would start to claim the much lower income replacement from Work and Income.

Compared to other OECD countries, New Zealand is in the group of countries with lower expenditure on active labour market programmes. In 2016, New Zealand spent 0.15% of its GDP on administering its employment service (Figure 5.4, Panel A) and a similar amount on actual employment supports and labour market programmes (Panel B). Within the latter spending group, the largest share goes to training measures and very little is spent for supported employment and vocational rehabilitation (again, Panel B).

Figure 5.4. New Zealand belongs to the group of OECD countries with relatively low spending on active labour market programmes and training

Expenditure on active labour market programmes, selected OECD countries, 2016, percentage of GDP

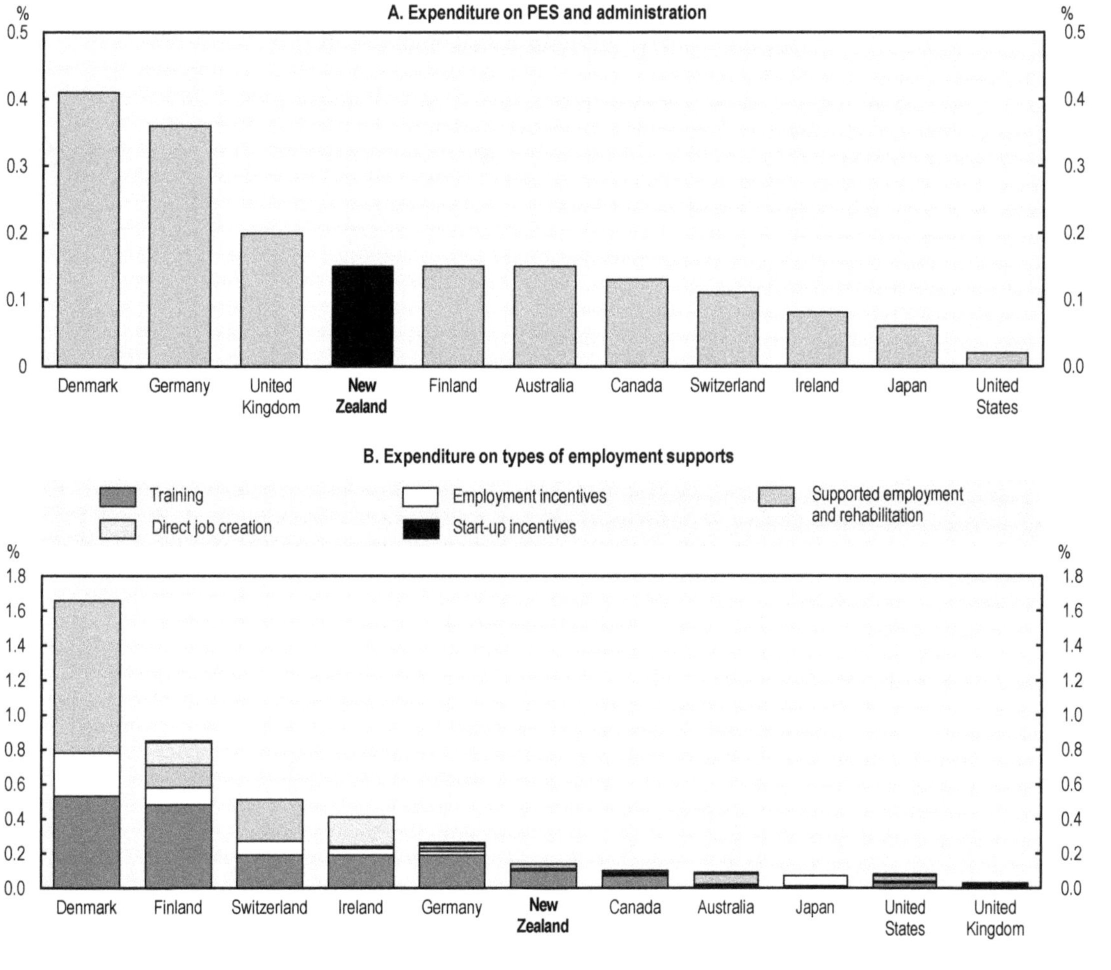

PES = Public Employment Service.

Source: OECD Labour Market Programme Database, https://stats.oecd.org/Index.aspx?QueryId=49447.

StatLink http://dx.doi.org/10.1787/888933845681

Benefit data underestimate the real number of people with mental health conditions

The figures on claims due to mental health conditions underestimate the *actual* number of people claiming benefits who have mental health conditions, as they only refer to people for whom a mental health condition is their primary reason for their claim. OECD analysis of 2014 data from the General Social Survey (GSS), found that 44% of people on JS-WR and 55% on JS-HCD met the criteria for a mental health condition.[3] This means that across the Jobseekers benefit population, the proportion of people meeting the criteria for a mental health condition is 48%, a much greater proportion than the 22% who are identified as claiming due to mental health conditions (Figure 5.5).

This data from the GSS also estimated that people with mental health conditions claiming SLP is higher, at 53% of all SLP claimants, while only 35% have a mental health condition as their primary reason for claiming (GSS, 2014). Furthermore, the GSS data identified that 49% of people claiming Sole Parent Support (SPS) met the criteria for a mental health condition. The same analysis was repeated using data from the New Zealand Health Survey 2016/2017, with similar results (Figure 5.5).[4]

Figure 5.5. Primary reason for benefits claims underestimates the proportion of people with mental health conditions on all main benefits

Share of people with a mental health condition on each type of income support

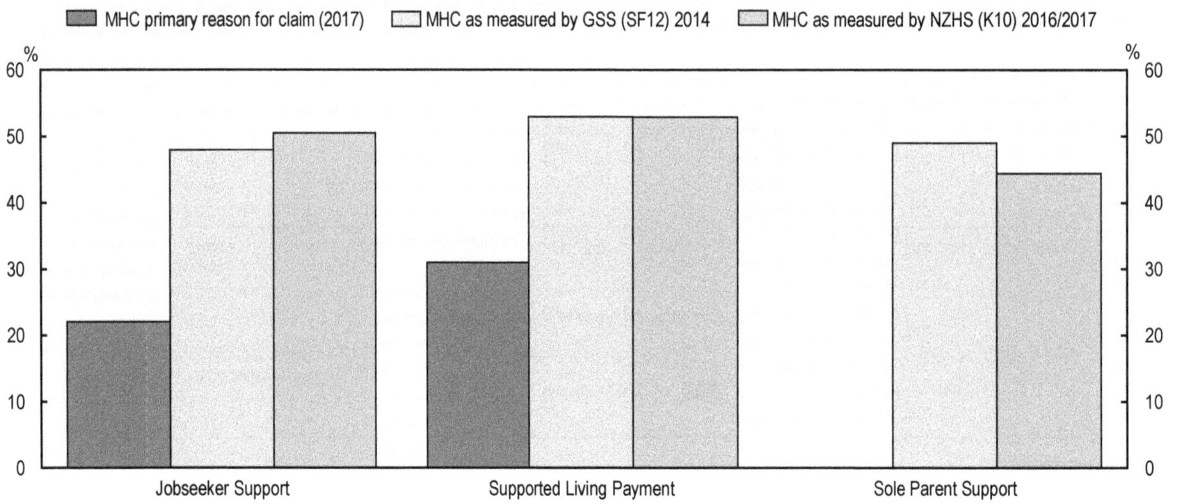

Note: MHC = Mental Health Condition.

Source: Secretariat estimates based on Ministry of Social Development, Benefits Tables, 2017; General Social Survey, 2014; and New Zealand Health Survey 2016/2017.

StatLink http://dx.doi.org/10.1787/888933845700

This underestimation of mental health need within the welfare population has significant implications for the provision of early and effective psychological and employment support (as discussed later in this chapter). It also highlights how important it is that some health information is collected on everyone claiming benefit, and that this is regularly reviewed, to ensure the right types and intensity of assistance can be provided.

One legislative obstacle in this is New Zealand's Privacy Act, which currently prohibits staff working within the social welfare system from accessing information on client health conditions if this is not a reason for claiming benefit. Given this legislative barrier, routinely screening everyone for mental health issues who claims benefit, becomes even more important (again, see the discussion later in this chapter).

The effectiveness of work capacity and support needs assessments is unclear

To prevent health and disability claims it is essential to have effective tools in place, which identify the work capacity, potential barriers to employment, and likely support needs of individuals at an early stage, and to make available early provision of medical and employment support as necessary. In New Zealand, whilst there is no specific tool for claimants with mental health conditions, the intended approach for all claimants is to assess work capacity rather than working from a medical diagnosis.

The Welfare Reforms brought in a new staged assessment process to identify ability to work for people with health conditions and disabilities. (For more information, see Box 5.1). For clients with a health condition, this includes a self-assessment and a medical certification both of which have a focus on what a person can do at work with appropriate supports and services.

The Self-Assessment Questionnaire is a four-page form completed by the individual, which the person takes to their appointment to discuss with a case manager. The person completes the self-assessment if they are making a claim for benefit due to a health or disability, so this is not a questionnaire completed by all MSD clients.

The Self-Assessment Questionnaire was developed based on stakeholder feedback on what information would be useful to collect and takes a strengths-based approach. The questionnaire also asks about a person's hobbies and interests, with the aim to identify their interest and skills. It asks about what work the person has done, what they would like to do in the future and what work they think they would be good at. There are also questions asking the person when they expect to return to work, if at all, and if they got a job, the type of workplace support they think they need. The final section asks the person to identify what types of things will help them get a job and stop them from getting a job. Data on the completion rates and utility of the Self-Assessment Questionnaire is not available.[5]

It is unclear how many MSD clients complete a self-assessment and how effective this is at matching people to the right type and intensity of health and employment support. Depending on how effective the self-assessment is at helping people access the right supports in a timely manner, it could be used for all MSD clients, regardless of the reason for their claim, built into a new allocation and navigation process.

The Work Capacity Medical Certificate is completed by a registered medical practitioner (which includes psychiatrists), a nurse practitioner (Jobseeker Support clients only), a midwife (for clients who are pregnant), or a dentist (for dental-related conditions). Psychologists or chiropractors cannot complete the medical certificate. The medical certificate asks the health practitioner about barriers/limitations to work related to the health condition or disability and for a diagnosis. The health practitioner must assess whether the person's capacity is likely to improve and allow them to take up full-time or part-time work with appropriate accommodation and support. The certificate must include information on the treatment and support that will help the person improve or manage their condition; on accommodation and support that could assist the person into suitable employment; and on the likely date on which the person is expected to be able to return to work. The information in the Work Capacity Medical Certificate is used, along with other information, to decide on a client's benefit entitlement and work obligations.

The critical role of the medical certificate highlights the importance of training and guidance to health professionals, particularly general practitioners, in understanding the interrelationship between mental health and work, managing the sickness certification consultation, and providing payment so that there is sufficient time for these consultations to be completed (see also the discussion in Chapter 2).

As with the self-assessment, it is important that the medical certifications provide information that can identify the right psychological and employment support a person would need in a timely manner. The effectiveness of the medical certificate in this regard should also be evaluated.

In cases where more information is needed than what has been provided by the self-assessment and the medical certificate, an independent Work Ability Assessment (WAA) is carried out to identify what work a client can do, and the support and services they need to gain and retain work. The assessment is undertaken by a suitably qualified health professional, such as a psychologist, occupational therapist or occupational nurse, who is experienced in assisting people into work.

The WAA covers all people claiming benefits due to a health condition and disability, inclusive of people with mental health conditions. Since its introduction and up to January 2018, of the 3 500 WAA conducted, about 1 000 were undertaken with people with mental health conditions. The numbers of people going through a WAA represents a very low proportion of MSD clients and an even lower proportion of people who are claiming for mental health reasons.

Whilst work capacity assessment is an important part of effective reform of the disability system, countries across the OECD have struggled to make the structural reforms to prevent increasing disability claims for people with mental health conditions (OECD, 2015[13]). It is clear that the same is the case for New Zealand.

The current system, whilst increasing support and resources to people with health conditions and disabilities, still has a much greater focus on other jobseekers.

Many not matched to the right type of case management and employment support

"Activation schemes need to start with an intake phase, where jobseekers are profiled to assign them to the appropriate target group" (OECD, 2015[13]). In New Zealand all jobseekers meet with Work and Income case managers to understand their individual circumstances. However, like many other OECD countries, New Zealand does not routinely screen for mental health issues. The first contact with the welfare system is an important opportunity for this to occur, so that prompt and early support can be offered. This is also the time to understand other potential barriers to employment and health and social care needs.

New Zealand needs to identify a more effective system to routinely screen for mental health issues. This can be based on validated instruments for all people claiming benefits and should be combined with appropriate follow-up supports and services (Liwowsky et al., 2009[14]). Any screening tool needs to be informed by cultural models of health and wellbeing, so that inequities of access to support and services do not increase.

The process of understanding an individuals' health status and circumstances, work capacity and barriers to re-employment could be a role carried out by a government or non-government provider. Identifying the right people and organisations to undertake this process is particularly important. For example, assessments for Māori claimants could be delivered by Māori assessors, using Māori models of practice and engagement, such as whānau ora. Inequities will continue if a universal approach is taken to assessment.

In Flanders, Belgium, at the moment of intake all job seekers are systematically assessed for issues which may be barriers to their employment. Information includes employment-specific competencies and qualifications as well as job-search behaviours, communication and social skills, disabilities and health conditions, including mental health problems. If a caseworker thinks there are more significant mental health issues, claimants can be referred to the public employment service's psychologist or an externally contracted employment centre specialising in in-depth multi-disciplinary screening. Where people are identified as having a need for greater assistance, they are referred to higher intensity employment support services. At any point, the guidance and support can be intensified depending on the needs of the person or the opinion of the case manager. At the latest, this would be after nine months of unemployment, and six months for people under age 26. At this point, an individual action plan is set up and intensive employment support started. People who have had mental health needs picked up through in-house or external screening receive specialised support in their job search, through government or contracted employment service providers (OECD, 2013[15]).

The OAG audit in 2014 identified that whilst the MSD had made good progress bringing in a case management approach, it does not yet serve people with high and complex needs well, and "greater collaboration with other agencies is needed" (OAG, 2014[3]).

At the same time as bringing in the new case management model, MSD brought in an actuarial model to evaluate the likelihood of long-term benefit dependency. The valuation is based on "what happened in the past to people with similar background, using 30 years of data on patterns of benefit receipt" (Productivity Commission, 2015[4]). This information informs the priorities for investment in case management and employment services. Clients likely to incur high and long-term costs have access to the most intensive front-line service. However, in practice it appears that the type of case management and employment assistance people are given predominantly depends on benefit they receive.

Jobseekers work-ready (JS-WR)

Within the current system people assessed as eligible for JS (work ready) would be allocated to work-search support case management (if they need additional support with job searching or work preparation activities) or general case management. Work-search support case managers have a caseload of 217 clients, and general case managers a caseload of 366 clients (OAG, 2014[3]). For the large numbers of people who have not had their mental health needs picked up, it is likely that these case management services will not be intensive enough to support them effectively. This group therefore faces a high risk of remaining unemployed or perhaps losing a new job again very quickly. During this time, they also face a greater risk of their mental health worsening.

Incorrect allocation to inappropriate employment assistance was found to be a problem in the Australian social protection system. Where people with mental health conditions had been triaged to more intensive employment assistance, the gap between their employment outcomes and people with no mental health condition was much smaller than for those who had been allocated to less intensive employment services. Jobseekers with mental health conditions were triaged into less intensive employment services largely because their mental health issues had not been identified as a barrier to employment at assessment (OECD, 2015[16]). While comparable research for New Zealand is unavailable, the setup and mechanisms are similar to those in Australia.

Jobseekers health condition or disability (JS-HCD)

The pathway is different for people claiming JS-HCD who are allocated to work-focused case management, if there is availability. Where caseloads are full, clients receive general case management services until availability of active case management services. Work-focused case management has a caseload of between 100 and 120 clients per case manager. The exception is young people aged 18-24 where caseloads are between 80 and 100 (OAG, 2014[3]). The caseload ratios for external providers appear to be lower and are likely to vary across providers. Where people have full exemptions from work obligations, the take up of employment assistance is voluntary. It is also likely that external providers also carry out a process for determining a person's employment assistance needs, which may be leading to duplication of assessment.

A process evaluation conducted at the time of the Health and Disability welfare reforms, examined the working partnership between Work and Income, a general practice and an external contracted provider in relation to people with a diagnosed mental health condition. At that time, supporting people on sickness-related benefits through case management was a new area for Work and Income. The evaluation identified that the first thing Work and Income case managers would do is to assess entitlement for financial support, while a conversation about work may or may not happen, depending on the person's health issues. If such conversation about work did not happen straightaway, it might happen at some point down the track when the case manager thinks the person is ready for work. The decision to refer the client to an external employment provider seemed to depend on whether a person needed more support than a Work and Income case manager could offer (Te Pou, 2013[17]).

Supported Living Payment

All people claiming SLP are allocated general case management services, as the focus is on administering their income support. People claiming SLP are not subject to work test obligations, but some may have work preparation obligations. People claiming SLP can opt in for work-focused case management, but only 0.5% of all SLP claimants do so. Not being in active case management will often mean not to be referred to the right level of service. However, SLP clients can access supported employment service irrespective of the level of case management.

Non-beneficiaries with mental health conditions

The allocation of employment services by benefit type also means that people who are not eligible for welfare benefits are not able to access Work and Income or contracted external provider employment support services. This would also include people at risk of losing their job due to mental health conditions. Non-beneficiaries appear only to be covered if Vote Health funding is paying for the employment support service, or if they are receiving vocational rehabilitation service through an ACC claim. There are examples of employment services funded through Vote Health within specialist mental health and addiction services (see Chapter 2). This is an area that needs to be prioritised and addressed, particularly for people with mental health conditions, in order to reduce personal hardship and later societal costs.

The logic of MSD's approach is to match case management intensity to the identified needs of the client (OAG, 2014[3]). However, if mental health needs are not picked up through contact with a Work and Income case manager, the actuarial allocation process will not be effective in matching people to the right type and intensity of employment assistance.

Figure 5.6 shows the various routes to case management and employment assistance by benefit type. The largest number of people is those claiming Sole Parent Support and JS-WR, of whom 50% will have a mental health issue; they are receiving either general case management or work-focused case management. While there are more options for people receiving benefits for mental health reasons, these are not available across all regions, and people have to opt-in for additional support.

Figure 5.6. The routes to case management and employment assistance by benefit type

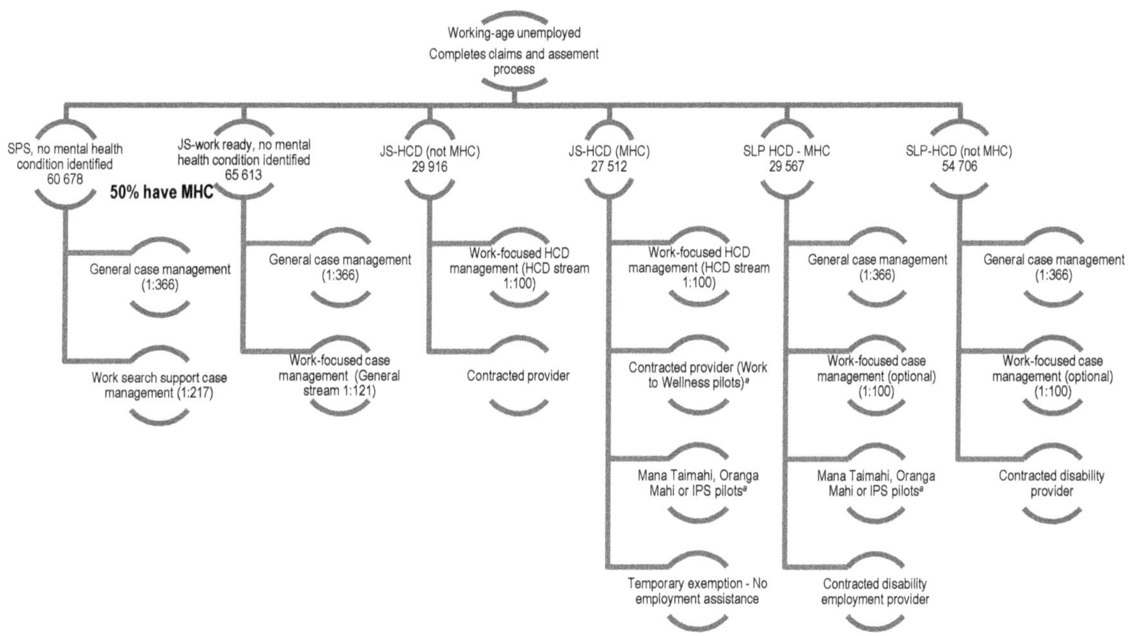

a) This initiative is currently a trial and is not available in every region/for all clients.
Source: Benefit claims figures taken from MSD Quarterly Benefits fact sheets, December, 2017.

It is also important to note that the logic of the actuarial allocation process is not applied in practice to people on SLP. In fact, the reverse seems to be the case in that people claiming SLP are allocated the least intensive general case management and can opt into more intensive work-focused case management. Even if a person opts-in, the assistance is unlikely to be intensive enough, although supported-employment programmes delivered by contracted providers may be available to offer more intense employment assistance.

It appears that a major issue effecting people with identified and unidentified mental health conditions is being allocated to inappropriate case management and employment support. This could lead to people going in and out of different advisors and providers (government and non-government) and through this process losing motivation and potentially getting further away from the labour market. It is also likely that their mental health will be deteriorating if they are not accessing the appropriate health services either.

A process evaluation of clients' experiences within and across case management and employment services, in 2013, highlighted the multiple assessment processes clients may go through, especially if information is incomplete or not passed on. This could happen between different case managers or between the work-focused case manager and the external service provider (Te Pou, 2013[17]).

One indication of the lack of early access to appropriate supports and services for this group is that 55% of new claims for SLP come from people previously claiming JS-HCD (administrative data supplied by MSD). Transfers from JS-HCD to SLP-HCD are also much higher than reverse transfers from SLP-HCD back to JS-HCD: 1 266 transfers per quarter compared to only 196 reverse transfers (Taylor-Fry, 2016). This implies that a frequent and well-trodden pathway for a jobseeker with a health condition or disability on JS-HCD is a gradual move into a generally permanent disability benefit.

MSD should also be monitoring the transfer from JS-WR to JS-HCD and the corresponding reverse transfer, in general and for people with mental health issues in particular, to better understand the impact of case management and employment assistance services.

For Māori and Pacific people claiming JS-HCD and SLP for mental health reasons, the pathway to de facto permanent disability benefits appears to be even more likely. Whilst data on transitions could not be examined by ethnicity, data on claimants by ethnicity show that the number of Māori and Pacific people claiming SLP for mental health reasons is increasing at a faster rate than for other ethnic groups.

Ethnic inequities highlight how important it is that case management and employment assistance are informed and designed by Māori and Pacific communities; otherwise, inequities will likely continue to worsen. For example, whānau ora plans could describe the narrative, which then helps to understand the contributing factors to being out of work. Whānau Ora wrap-around support services would be case management approaches that are inclusive of whānau and describe a narrative of the presenting issues of concern, and the solutions. MSD has adopted one such model, Te Whare Tapa Wha in its Intensive Client Support trials (see Box 2.3 in Chapter 2).

Given these inequities, it is strongly recommended that future actuarial reports continue to monitor the experience of people claiming benefits for mental health reasons and that this is expanded to include an analysis of benefit inflows and off-flows as well as benefits transfers by ethnicity and other socio-demographic characteristics.

The welfare reforms also brought a greater focus on work obligations, with 80 000 more people now having such obligations (OAG, 2014[3]). At December 2017, 70% of all working-age adults on benefits had work obligations (201 874 people with work obligations out of 289 788 total recipients), with most people receiving either JS or Sole Parent Support. If people do not comply with their work obligations, sanctions can be imposed. About 15 000 sanctions are imposed each quarter, of which approximately 3 000 per quarter result in benefits suspension or cancellation. About two in three sanctions are for missed appointments (OAG, 2017[5]). Data from the December 2017 shows that 42% of imposed sanctions were for Māori and 11% for Pacific clients. The Auditor-General, in 2014, made a number of recommendations to MSD on how to reduce missed appointments, including reminding people through text messaging, and encouraging innovative practice to increase the percentage of appointments kept. Again, ensuring the use of Māori-led models of care and support and involving whānau could potentially help to understand and reduce the number of missed appointments of Māori clients.[6]

In addition to varying across benefit type, the current case management procedure and corresponding outcomes appear to vary across the country as well. It is important for MSD to collect data on regional practices and performance in a systematic manner and to introduce appropriate feedback mechanisms to ensure that laggard regions can learn from vanguard regions and thus ensure better overall outcomes.

Early evaluation of the recent welfare reforms found that work-focused case management was effective at supporting sole parents into work. As a result, MSD added another 18 000 sole parents to the work-focused case management stream (OAG, 2014[3]). Given the reforms have not been as successful for people with mental health conditions, the expansion in case management for this group has not taken place in the same way. This is understandable and likely to be explained at least for some of the client group by a lack of well-integrated employment and health services. Any obstacles to better employment outcomes should be removed; this could include strengthening work-focused case management and building the capacity of both the employment and health sectors to be more aware of and responsive to the interrelationship between mental health and work.

The New Zealand social protection system needs to improve the approach it takes to the identification of individual employment assistance needs. Whilst some MSD clients appear to be receiving the appropriate level and intensity of employment support, the vast majority are not. The system is therefore missing the opportunity to provide the right support, at the right time, and reduce the flow of people onto health and disability benefits.

There is a lack of funding for and access to psychological support

OECD countries' social protection systems can address clients' health needs by either co-ordinating its services with the health care system or providing integrated health services as part of the social protection system. Sweden, for example has pooled resources between its national employment service, the regional health authority and welfare offices, and its national social insurance scheme (OECD, 2013[18]).

In New Zealand, psychological support is not routinely offered to MSD clients. A doctor, usually a GP, can however provide the necessary information to case managers to authorise the use of Disability Allowance payments for counselling, for some people. The allowance covers ten sessions initially, which must be provided through a counsellor with recognised qualifications. Health practitioners and members of the New Zealand Association of Counsellors or the Social Workers Registration Board can provide such counselling support. People can apply for additional sessions. At March 2018, 1 139 clients were accessing counselling using a Disability Allowance. The majority (92%) were people claiming benefits for mental health reasons; 16% of the total identified as Māori, 2% as Pacific, and 62% as NZ European. Counselling not related to a person's disability or health condition, such as relationship counselling, is not financially reimbursed.

Work and Income employs Health and Disability Advisors to provide advice to case managers, regional leadership teams and the national office. There are 39 such advisors working across New Zealand, nine in Auckland and three in each of the other ten Work and Income regions, plus one principal health adviser and one principal disability advisor to support the regional health and disability advisors and ensure a nationally consistent approach is being taken. None of these advisors can provide psychological treatment.

Health and Disability Advisors have a variety of health and disability backgrounds. Some are trained psychologists, others have backgrounds as social workers, employment advisors, rehabilitation experts or mental health nurses. All advisors have completed Mental Health 101 (MH101).

Anecdotal reports suggest people outside the welfare system, particularly in the medical services, find it hard to get information from Work and Income, terming the system a black hole. A small-scale evaluation identified one-way communication between general practitioners and Work and Income staff, where health professionals will send a letter to Work and Income but will not get a response unless there is consent from the client or the GP has formal authority to act as an advocate for the client (Te Pou, 2013[17]).

The Social Security Act allows for limited communication around the purpose for which the external agency is involved. For example, when a doctor fills out a medical certificate and this information is sent to Work and Income, the latter can communicate directly with the doctor to seek clarification around the information provided. If additional information is required, such as a specialist report, separate specific client consent is needed. MSD advises to involve in such situations Health and Disability Advisors who usually have an established relationship with the health professional. The guidance for the case managers therefore is to seek advice from the Health and Disability Advisors rather than contact the doctor. If needed, Work and Income can have case conferences involving general practitioners and specialists.

Expand the current approach to building case workers' mental health competences

Across the OECD, mental health competencies and psychological expertise in the employment sector are underdeveloped and not commensurate with the high prevalence of mental health issues among jobseekers and welfare clients. Better mental health competencies need to be developed to make early identification and quick intervention possible in all systems. Efforts in that direction should come primarily in the unemployment system because better job retention and reintegration at this early stage can prevent people with poor mental health from slipping into welfare and disability.

It is important therefore that all front-line Work and Income staff receive training, which builds their mental health competence, cultural competency and psychological expertise. MSD currently invests in different training courses to build mental health competencies of staff (see Table 5.4). Immediate post-training evaluation of the available training shows that the courses are having the desired impact. However, evidence has shown that any training needs to be following up by practice and support in a person's everyday working context, in order for the learning to be sustained (Fixsen et al., 2005[19]).

Whilst awareness training and the recognition of signs of mental distress, are a crucial step, this should be built upon so that Work and Income staff not only develop the skills to identify mental health issues, but decide when to seek support from specialists, and where such support can be found. This is an area where improvement is needed for most OECD countries. Training should help Work and Income staff understand the interrelationship between mental health and work, and the impact of mental health conditions on work capacity. This is because staff working in the benefits system frequently underestimates the work capacity of people with mental health conditions (OECD, 2015[13]).

Table 5.4. There are a range of mental health competency training sessions for MSD staff

Course name	Duration	Aims	Reach	Evaluation
Lives Like Mine	2.5 hours	The importance of empathy to enhance positive outcomes for MSD clients.	4 692 staff trained Applies to all MSD staff	1 300 staff completed the post session evaluation. **96%** of respondents agreed with the statement *"I have a better understanding of how my actions and values can influence client outcomes."* **95%** of respondents agreed with the statement *"I have a greater level of self-awareness of what might be going on in the lives of others (i.e. my colleagues or clients)."* **99%** of respondents agreed with the statement *"I intend to continue to reflect on how my attitudes and behaviours may impact on what I do in my job."*
Mental Health 101	One day	To build confidence to recognise, relate and respond to people experiencing mental health issues.	3 419 staff trained	An evaluation of 13 MH101 workshops found that: A **56%** increase in confidence of recognising signs and symptoms of mental health conditions. A **65%** increase in confidence in knowing how to respond
Suicide Awareness	3.5 hours	How to recognise and respond to people at risk of suicide.	1 731 (of expected 4 000) trained	476 staff completed the pre-workshop evaluation and 807 have completed the post-workshop evaluation. Participants were asked *"what is your confidence level in being able to identify someone at risk of suicide?"* Prior to the workshop staff confidence levels were at **34**%, and this increased significantly to **85%** post workshop. Learners also expressed feeling more confident about holding an effective conversation with someone who is having suicidal thoughts – **39**% of staff were confident pre-workshop, which has risen to **84**% post-workshop.
Work to Wellness	90 minutes (online)	Supporting clients diagnosed with a mental health condition who have part-time, deferred or no work obligations.	502 staff trained Targeted at WFCMs	N/A
Lives Like Mine Outtakes	3 hours	An extension of Lives Like Mine, a focus on case studies and increasing self-awareness	N/A	Over 550 staff completed the post-session evaluation. **94%** of respondents agreed or were neutral with the statement *"I feel confident to apply my new knowledge and skills from the training to my role."* **93%** of respondents agreed or were neutral with the statement *"This training has helped me to further develop and improve what I do in my job."*
Rethinking Mental Health	5x one-hour modules	Explores the experiences people with mental health conditions may have had and encourages effective engagement from front line staff.	N/A	512 staff complete the post session evaluation **95%** of respondents agreed or were neutral with the statement *"I felt I understood why I was doing this learning programme before starting and how it would benefit me."* **98%** of respondents agreed or were neutral with the statement *"I feel confident to apply my new knowledge and skills from the training to my role."* **95%** of respondents agreed or were neutral with the statement *"This training has helped me to further develop and improve what I do in my job."*

Source: Data supplied from Ministry of Social Development, April 2018.

It is also not clear how much access case managers get to training in psychological techniques, like brief interventions. Whilst they can access advice from the Health and Disability Advisor, there are only 19 such advisors across the country.

MSD should ensure supervision builds on the training provided and helps staff to identify mental health issues, as well as other health barriers to work, including addiction and physical health issues. Case managers need to know how clients can access appropriate, specialist support locally. It is also essential that all trainings integrate cultural competency with mental health competency. For example, Work and Income staff need to know how to facilitate whānau hui and engagement with Māori whānau and should also be supported to seek out cultural supervision to talk through case-specific situations.

It is also essential that Work and Income staff represent the cultural diversity of the communities with which they work. Given the overrepresentation of Māori people claiming welfare benefits, MSD should review the profile of Māori case managers and seek to recruit more Māori case managers as needed.

Mental health and employment services are in their fifth year of piloting

Employment and health needs are rarely addressed together. Even where jobseekers' mental health issues are recognised, people are often plainly exempted from job-search and availability requirements and expected to seek treatment until they return fit and healthy to seek work. This is evident in the New Zealand welfare system although it is an approach found not to be effective (OECD, 2015[13]).

Delivering co-ordinated, integrated health and employment services is challenging because of the lack of coherent incentives, obligations and guidelines for stakeholders and participating professionals. Integrating services requires public employment services to address clients' health and employment needs concurrently. Funding and policy mechanisms are needed which stimulate cooperation between employment services (government and non-government) and the health sector, especially primary and community-based mental health services.

In 2013, MSD started to examine this need for coordinated, integrated health and employment services. A tender process was run to select and contract with external providers to deliver employment support services to people in receipt of JS-HCD with a mental health diagnosis. These Mental Health and Employment Service (MHES) pilots were then run for three years, in four regions of the country.

In 2016, following an evaluation conducted by MSD, the MHES pilots were replaced by Work to Wellness (W2W) pilots and a new tender process announced. W2W pilots cover the same target group as MHES pilots, people on JS-HCD with a mental health diagnosis who are interested in finding work. Providers are contracted by MSD to deliver outcomes-based case management, placement and post-placement support. Providers are paid for full-time and part-time employment outcomes, as well as job retention milestones. W2W contracts aimed to improve on MHES by 1) improving the links to health services to help the integration of mental health treatment into employment services; 2) defining client outcomes in broader terms; and 3) decreasing the dropout rates. W2W services are available in the same four regions as MHES, plus a fifth region, and aim to provide employment support for 2 000 clients for two years. There are currently more than 200 clients enrolled. A formal evaluation of W2W is currently underway, and a report is expected later in 2018. Early findings suggest that W2W pilots are experiencing challenges getting the right type of employment service to the right person at the right time, in reducing early exits and in integrating employment services with health provision. Whilst W2W aimed to increase the integration with health services, it appears the contracts may not have encouraged or recognised this.

W2W contracts pay providers an initial enrolment fee for each person accepted into their service meeting the eligibility criteria, a monthly activity fee per client, and further on payments based on job placements and successful job retention, at six and 12 months. Higher payments are received for clients with higher needs and for full-time employment.

If outcomes for these contracts are disappointing, it may be that payments to providers were too low, or the contract duration too short for the provider to make a real investment, or there may have been issues inherent in the contracting process, or the contract terms and conditions. Anecdotal evidence suggest that many of the external providers working with people on JS-HCD experience significant challenges getting referrals from Work and Income. All these potential issues should be investigated.

As at December 2017, MSD also funds 32 employment services that support people with disabilities and people with health conditions to gain and retain open employment, through contracting with external employment providers. Of these, six providers with a total service volume of approximately 680 people, specialise in supporting people with mental health conditions. These providers would predominantly be working with people whose mental health conditions is having a significant impact on their daily living, and likely to be claiming SLP. A new outcome-based payment system similar to that being used in W2W contracts, and a Service Level Intensity (SLI) rating system have recently been introduced under these National Supported Employment contracts. This is a step away from the old one-size-fits-all approach towards a more nuanced basis for aligning funding with the actual support needs of individuals. Anecdotal reports suggest that these contracted providers use whānau links, other community supports, health professionals, and other social services for their main referral pathways, rather than Work and Income case management. Although NZDSN are trialling a desk-based service profile tool, to provide information to case managers on their local disability providers.

New pilots aim at higher take up of case management and employment assistance

At the same time, MSD has set up a number of additional pilots for people with health conditions, including but not specifically for mental health conditions. These *Oranga Mahi* pilots are running across four district health boards. An investment of NZD 24 million supports these trials over three years. Evaluation of these trials is currently underway (OAG, 2017[5]).

One of these pilots is *Mana Taimahi*, an initiative co-designed and delivered with the National Hauora Coalition (NHC).[7] The main objective of Mana Taimahi is to support clients receiving Jobseeker Support with a health condition or disability into work, by testing new approaches to working with general practitioners. People on SLP are not eligible. The initial referral is made by GPs, who can promote *Mana Taimahi* to clients meeting the criteria at work-capacity medical certification consultations.

Mana Taimahi began as a Proof of Concept (POC) that ran between August 2016 and June 2017, involving two general practices and two community links in West Auckland. The POC was designed because in talking with GPs they found that:

- The limited interaction between GPs and case managers with mutual clients has resulted in misunderstandings about Work and Income services and processes and the work abilities of JS-HCD clients;
- Time pressures on GP appointments and limited information about how to support clients to return to work, mean that GPs struggle to offer work-focused support to patients who need it.

The *Mana Taimahi* POC confirmed that the apparent disconnect between Work and Income and GPs can contribute to sustained periods on benefit for mutual clients, which can also have a negative impact on health. The POC aimed to address these issues through education modules for GPs, networking meetings between GPs and Work and Income case managers, and free GP visits for clients on JS-HCD. Anecdotal reports have found that the feedback from the GPs has been very positive. They feel the trial has made a difference to their knowledge and perception of services and brought them in a much better space to support clients into work.

The *Mana Taimahi* POC resulted in 57% of clients being referred to MSD related programmes and providers, while 20% have entered employment. This is a group of clients able to choose to opt into MSD programmes and support services; a step that many of them, however, would usually avoid.

The POC is currently scaled up to a prototype to test the concept on a larger scale. The prototype will run from November 2017 to November 2018 continuing the services established through the POC. In particular, it will aim to:

- help GPs to understand the negative health impacts of long-term unemployment, the health and social benefits of work, and the misconceptions about Work and Income services;
- provide up to three additional free GP consultations for clients to allow GPs to have in-depth discussions with clients about their wider circumstances, their employment goals and the appropriate steps needed for them to return to work;
- hold regular meetings between GPs and Work and Income staff to improve communication, create a stronger understanding of one another's services, and ensure consistency of support for clients.

The *Mana Taimahi* approach, working directly with primary care teams, is a similar approach adopted by a mental health non-government provider. Employment support services have been co-located with general practice primary care teams to support people with mental health conditions to get and keep employment. These small-scale pilots were self-funded or utilised existing funding contracts from the Ministry of Health or the Ministry of Social Development. They provided one full-time employment advisor to two to three general practice teams. Evaluation of these pilots have found that general practitioners value the service and it also increased the frequency of employment-focused consultations held by the general practice teams (Te Pou, 2013[17]; Te Pou, 2013[20]). On average, these embedded primary care pilots support about 50% of people accepted onto the programme into employment.

MSD has also recently initiated funding for two services to trial the Individual Placement and Support (IPS) approach (see Chapter 2). The pilots are for 18-35 year olds diagnosed with a severe mental health condition (Auckland) and youth aged 16-24 years with mild-to-moderate mental health condition (Christchurch). To date, IPS services in New Zealand have been funded exclusively by money from Vote Health.

Social bonds are used in other OECD countries to support the delivery of integrated health and employment services.[8] The first social bond in New Zealand commissioned in 2017 aims at improving employment outcomes for people with mental health conditions who are on a welfare payment. A financial incentive is offered to a consortium of providers and investors if they can achieve a result with a service, which is demonstrably better than what has been previously achieved with the old way of doing things. The aim is to assist up to 1 700 people in South Auckland over the 60-month period of the bond. Under the contract terms, the employment service provider is allowed six months from referral to finding people a job. Therapeutic help is also delivered, where needed. Once a job has been found, people can be supported for up to two years to help them remain in work. Intermediate results from the social bonds contract, however, seem to be disappointing. Every effort will have to be made to understand the reasons to strengthen the contract and to ensure better outcomes in any future contract.

In conclusion, there are a range of promising programmes, pilots and experiments available, but these remain limited in scale and regions. Furthermore, most of these programmes and pilots are not available to people who are non-beneficiaries, with the exception of the health-funded IPS programmes. Rigorous independent evaluation is needed of all programmes and pilots so that findings can inform future contracting.

Annual appropriations for MSD to cover contracted-out services are around NZD 41 million. This compares with costs of in-house case management and work broker services worth around NZD 240 million. A further NZD 307 million covers the administration of income support (Productivity Commission, 2015[4]). Therefore, contracted-out services represent a very small proportion of MSD's total investments in the provision of case management and employment services.

Pilots that integrate health and employment services need scaling up

Easy and early access to employment support services appears to be a significant issue. Many specialist employment support services are only available to people with a diagnosed mental health conditions, or people on certain types of benefits, or only if the person is referred through the Work and Income case manager, or only in some parts of the country. Furthermore, all employment support services that specialise in working with people with mental health conditions are on time-limited service contracts, which makes recruiting and retaining an adequate workforce challenging.

The pilots working directly with general practice teams are bringing employment support much earlier, rather than waiting for a referral from a Work and Income case manager. They are also serving as a bridge between the client and Work and Income offering navigation support to apply for financial support and other social services.

There is an urgent need to have national access to evidence-based vocational interventions for jobseekers with mental health conditions, which combine psychological counselling with pre- and post-placement services, learning from successful pilots that have combined employment support with improved communication between Work and Income case managers and health practitioners.

Of note is that the audit-general's report from 2014 notes that "International evidence on successful outcomes for people with multiple barriers to employment is limited, and the Ministry might need to build its own evidence base to find out what work". This is a potentially misleading statement partly explaining the lack of scale-up of employment services since the science of vocational rehabilitation for people facing multiple barriers to employment is an area of psychosocial rehabilitation, which has advanced significantly over the past 30 years (Drake and Bond, 2017[21]).

It is important that pilots are informed by existing evidence, including Māori models of practice. The issue lies less in trying to work out "what works", as there is good evidence for that, but in ensuring the authorising system can enable good practice to be implemented. Experience with MHES and W2W contracts is perhaps an illustration of this issue. The contracts were changed, but on the ground their appears still to be an issue of getting integrated health and employment services or reducing drop-out rates.

A recent policy analysis, which investigated the strengths and weaknesses of MOH and MSD contracts and the contracting process, concluded the current contracting environment is hindering not assisting the labour force participation of people with mental health conditions. There are many purchasers, each with different types of contracts, and an uncoordinated approach to contracting and purchasing across government agencies. The analysis recommended identifying a lead agency for coordinating health and welfare policy in relation to purchasing employment services for people with mental health conditions and starting a trial of pooled investment. The analysis also recommended amending the fee structures to reward job tenure over hours of employment, encouraging post-placement support and better specifying and rewarding closer integration between health and employment services and alignment with evidence-based practices (Lockett, Waghorn and Kydd, 2018[22]).

Whilst these issues were raised in the context of the labour force disadvantage of people experiencing mental health conditions, they echo the findings from the 2015 New Zealand Productivity Commission's more effective social services report. This review of New Zealand's social services also focused on improvements that need to be made to the authorising systems, particularly the purchasing and contracting environment (Productivity Commission, 2015[4]). The government has responsibility for good systems stewardship and the creation of an enabling environment for social services to operate effectively within and this is especially important for people who have higher or more complex needs, who are affected the most by the silo nature of much of the available service funding, purchasing and delivery.

New guidelines for providers of employment support services for people with disabilities have recently been launched (NZDSN, 2018[23]). These could provide a quality benchmark for (government and non-government) employment support providers, and adherence to these guidelines built into contracts and quality management processes, along with known evidence-based practices in employment support services, like the Individual Placement and Support fidelity scale. This could sit alongside contracts that reward providers for integrating with health services, providing early intervention, and providing post-placement support. Consideration should be given to the best contracting environment to enable what works, to be implemented in the New Zealand context, and to assist with scaling-up of successful pilots.

Conclusion

In 2011, a Welfare Working Group set out a set of practical recommendations to reduce long-term welfare dependency for people of working age, their families and the wider community. Within this report the Group highlighted the fact that "gaps in mental health, rehabilitation and managed-care services create costs which inevitably show in the welfare system, not to mention costs to individuals in terms of their well-being"; and that "joblessness is particularly harmful to mental and physical health". At that time, 41% of people receiving the then Sickness Benefit and 29% of people receiving the then Invalid's Benefit had mental health conditions as their primary reason for claiming. The Group called for specialist employment interventions to support people with mental health conditions to work, and a greater investment in psychological therapies.

The structural and operational reforms since the Welfare Working Group report have had minimal impact on people with mental health conditions. In fact, the numbers of people with mental health conditions claiming benefits is increasing, particularly for Māori and Pacific people. There are also many people claiming welfare benefits whose mental health issues are not formally recognised by the welfare system; conditions that may not be the assessed cause for the benefit claim but still pose a major barrier to re-employment. As a result, the supports and services offered for many are not effectively matching their needs for employment assistance. Even where mental health needs are recognised, there is limited access to timely and appropriate treatment and employment assistance.

There is no focus in the New Zealand welfare system on early intervention for people with mental health conditions, and more generally. For people who are off sick from work or not employed and not claiming welfare benefits, there is virtually no employment assistance available. Addressing this issue is of paramount importance and will need significant cross-government collaboration.

New pilots aim to support people with mental health conditions to access Work and Income case management and employment assistance, or employment assistance from a contracted provider. These new pilots recognise the need to integrate health and employment services. This is a promising development, but these are available to a tiny proportion of the population in need of these services. Well-integrated health and employment support services should be scaled up and the findings from promising pilots translated into lasting and structural reform.

Finally, there is a need for more effective assessment and more timely access to appropriate support including integrated psychological and employment support services. The current pathway to early and appropriate employment assistance and psychological support is unclear, inconsistent and inequitable.

Notes

[1] A recently established Welfare Expert Advisory Group will advise the government on changes to obligations and associated sanctions applied to beneficiaries to ensure alignment with the vision of the new government. In practice, sanctions are not often applied.

[2] NZDSN is the New Zealand Disability Support Network, a network of NGOs that provide support services for people with disabilities. The purpose of the Network is to lead and influence change that supports inclusive lives for people with disabilities.

[3] The General Social Survey uses the Short Form Health Survey 12 item scale (SF-12), which measures the impact of mental health on role functioning.

[4] The New Zealand Health Survey uses the Kessler Psychological Distress 10 item scale (K-10), to measure levels of psychological distress in the past 4 weeks.

[5] The Self-Assessment Questionnaire is not linked to a person's claims process; hence, it is not used to decide on benefit entitlements.

[6] A forthcoming report by the Welfare Expert Advisory Group will reconsider obligations in the welfare system and associated sanctions imposed.

[7] The National Hauora Coalition is a Māori-led and culturally driven Primary Health Organisation focused on improving outcomes for all whānau.

[8] Social Bonds are a method of providing health and social services, where upfront-funding is provided by private investors. If the agreed outcomes are reached, the government pays back the investor a pre-determined return on the investment. The following link provides an example: https://www.socialfinance.org.uk/projects/health-and-employment-partnerships-hep.

References

Drake, R. and G. Bond (2017), "Individual Placement and Support: Penetration and New Populations", *Administration and Policy in Mental Health and Mental Health Services Research*, Vol. 44/3, pp. 309-310, http://dx.doi.org/10.1007/s10488-017-0803-4. [21]

Fixsen, D. et al. (2005), *Implementation Research: A Synthesis of the Literature*, University of South Florida, Tampa, https://nirn.fpg.unc.edu/sites/nirn.fpg.unc.edu/files/resources/NIRN-MonographFull-01-2005.pdf (accessed on 29 October 2018). [19]

Greenfield, A., H. Miller and G. Mcguire (2016), *Ministry of Social Development: Valuation of the Benefit System for Working-age Adults*, Taylor Fry Pty Ltd - Consulting Actuaries & Analytics Professionals, Sydney, http://www.taylorfry.com.au (accessed on 29 October 2018). [6]

Liwowsky, I. et al. (2009), "Screening for depression in the older long-term unemployed", *Social Psychiatry and Psychiatric Epidemiology*, Vol. 44/8, pp. 622-627, http://dx.doi.org/10.1007/s00127-008-0478-y. [14]

Lockett, H., G. Waghorn and R. Kydd (2018), "Policy barriers to evidence-based practices in vocational rehabilitation for people with psychiatric disabilities in New Zealand", *Work*, Vol. Preprint/Preprint, pp. 1-14, http://dx.doi.org/10.3233/WOR-182752. [22]

MSD (2018), *Benefit Fact Sheets Ministry of Social Development*, Ministry of Social Development, Wellington, http://www.msd.govt.nz (accessed on 26 July 2018). [7]

MSD (2018), *Benefit rates at 1 April 2018 - Work and Income*, https://www.workandincome.govt.nz/products/benefit-rates/benefit-rates-april-2018.html (accessed on 29 October 2018). [24]

MSD (2017), *2017 Benefit fact sheets archive*, Benefit fact sheets archive, https://www.msd.govt.nz/about-msd-and-our-work/publications-resources/statistics/benefit/archive-2017.html (accessed on 29 October 2018). [8]

MSD (2014), *Working differently with people with health conditions, mental health conditions and disabilities to assist them into work - Ministry of Social Development*, https://www.msd.govt.nz/about-msd-and-our-work/publications-resources/research/welfare-reform-health-disability/working-differently-with-people-with-health-conditions.html (accessed on 26 July 2018). [9]

New Zealand Productivity Commission (2015), *More effective social services*, ew Zealand Productivity Commission, Wellington, https://www.productivity.govt.nz/sites/default/files/social-services-final-report-main.pdf (accessed on 30 June 2018). [26]

NZDSN (2018), *Employment Support Practice Guidelines*, New Zealand Disability Support Network, Wellington, https://www.nzdsn.org.nz/wp-content/uploads/2018/03/F_7270-NZD_Employment_Guidelines_WEB.pdf (accessed on 29 October 2018). [23]

NZDSN (2016), *Transformation, Inclusion and Citizenship*, New Zealand Disability Support Network, Wellington, https://www.nzdsn.org.nz/wp-content/uploads/2016/08/NZDSN_Transformation-Inclusion-and-Citizenship_v8-FINAL-2-08-2016.pdf (accessed on 29 October 2018). [10]

NZDSN (2015), *Investing for Innovation and Quality*, New Zealand Disability Support Network , Wellington, https://www.nzdsn.org.nz/wp-content/uploads/2016/03/NZDSN-Sector_Briefing-28_July_2015.pdf (accessed on 29 October 2018). [11]

OAG (2017), *Ministry of Social Development: Using a case management approach to service delivery - Progress in responding to the Auditor-General's recommendations*, Office of the Auditor-General, Wellington, https://www.oag.govt.nz/2017/msd-follow-up/docs/msd-case-management.pdf (accessed on 29 October 2018). [5]

OAG (2014), *Ministry of Social Development: Using a case management approach to service delivery*, Office of the Auditor-General, Wellington, https://oag.govt.nz/2014/msd-case-management/docs/msd-case-management.pdf (accessed on 29 October 2018). [3]

ODI (2016), *New Zealand Disability Strategy 2016-2026*, Office for Disability Issues, Wellington, https://www.odi.govt.nz/assets/New-Zealand-Disability-Strategy-files/pdf-nz-disability-strategy-2016.pdf (accessed on 29 October 2018). [12]

OECD (2015), *Fit Mind, Fit Job: From evidence to practice in mental health and work.*, OECD Publishing, Paris. [13]

OECD (2015), *Mental Health and Work: Australia*, Mental Health and Work, OECD Publishing, Paris, http://dx.doi.org/10.1787/9789264246591-en. [16]

OECD (2015), *Recommendation of the Council on Integrated Mental Health, Skills and Work Policy*, OECD Publications, Paris, https://legalinstruments.oecd.org/Instruments/ShowInstrumentView.aspx?InstrumentID=334&Lang=en&Book=False (accessed on 08 February 2018). [25]

OECD (2013), *Mental Health and Work: Belgium*, Mental Health and Work, OECD Publishing, Paris, http://dx.doi.org/10.1787/9789264187566-en. [15]

OECD (2013), *Mental Health and Work: Sweden*, Mental Health and Work, OECD Publishing, Paris, http://dx.doi.org/10.1787/9789264188730-en. [18]

Productivity Commission (2015), *More effective social services*, New Zealand Productivity Commission, Wellington, https://www.productivity.govt.nz/sites/default/files/social-services-final-report-summary-version.pdf (accessed on 28 October 2018). [4]

Public Services Advisory Group (2011), *Better Public Services Advisory Group Report - November 2011*, State Services Commission, New Zealand Government, http://www.ssc.govt.nz/sites/all/files/bps-report-nov2011_0.pdf (accessed on 29 October 2018). [1]

Te Pou (2013), *A demonstration of integrated employment support in primary care*, Te Pou o te Whakaaro Nui, Auckland, https://www.tepou.co.nz/uploads/files/resource-assets/a-demonstration-of-integrated-employment-support-in-primary-care-formative-evaluation-report.pdf (accessed on 29 October 2018). [20]

Te Pou (2013), *Process evaluation of employment support in Wellington general practices*, Te Pou o te Whakaaro Nui, Auckland, https://www.tepou.co.nz/uploads/files/resource-assets/process-evaluation-of-employment-support-in-Wellington-general-practices.pdf (accessed on 29 October 2018). [17]

Work and Income (2013), *Overview of Welfare Reform July 2013 changes*, Work and Income, Wellington, http://www.workandincome.govt.nz (accessed on 29 October 2018). [2]

ORGANISATION FOR ECONOMIC CO-OPERATION AND DEVELOPMENT

The OECD is a unique forum where governments work together to address the economic, social and environmental challenges of globalisation. The OECD is also at the forefront of efforts to understand and to help governments respond to new developments and concerns, such as corporate governance, the information economy and the challenges of an ageing population. The Organisation provides a setting where governments can compare policy experiences, seek answers to common problems, identify good practice and work to co-ordinate domestic and international policies.

The OECD member countries are: Australia, Austria, Belgium, Canada, Chile, the Czech Republic, Denmark, Estonia, Finland, France, Germany, Greece, Hungary, Iceland, Ireland, Israel, Italy, Japan, Korea, Latvia, Lithuania, Luxembourg, Mexico, the Netherlands, New Zealand, Norway, Poland, Portugal, the Slovak Republic, Slovenia, Spain, Sweden, Switzerland, Turkey, the United Kingdom and the United States. The European Union takes part in the work of the OECD.

OECD Publishing disseminates widely the results of the Organisation's statistics gathering and research on economic, social and environmental issues, as well as the conventions, guidelines and standards agreed by its members.

OECD PUBLISHING, 2, rue André-Pascal, 75775 PARIS CEDEX 16
(81 2018 77 1 P) ISBN 978-92-64-30730-8 – 2018

www.ingramcontent.com/pod-product-compliance
Ingram Content Group UK Ltd.
Pitfield, Milton Keynes, MK11 3LW, UK
UKHW051503290926
15471UKWH00008B/1377

9 789264 307308